114

Youth Football Plays

Scott Tappa

Iola-Scandinavia Pee Wee Athletics

© 2019 Scott Tappa. All rights reserved.

No part of this book may be reproduced, stored in a retrieval system or transmitted, in any form or by any means, electronic, mechanical, photocopying, recording, or otherwise, without prior permission of Scott Tappa

Cover photos: Jana Tappa

Interior photos: Jana Tappa, Danielle Taggart, Steven Soik

scott_tappa@hotmail.com

twitter.com/scotttappa

youtube.com/scotttappa

firsttimecoach.blogspot.com

facebook.com/isfirebirds

To Dad, who showed me why kids need coaches

To Mom, who inspired a love of books and reading

To Jana, who created the perfect environment for coaches

To Will and Charlie, who made me a coach

*To all of the kids I've coached and guys I've coached with —
once a Firebird, always a Firebird*

TABLE OF CONTENTS

Dedication 5

Introduction 8

Offense Overview 12

Play Names 14

Lead Series 15

Pitch Series 50

Quick Series 64

Keeper Series 84

Rocket Series 98

Twins Series 108

Trips Series 120

Empty Series 128

Defense 134

Special Teams 138

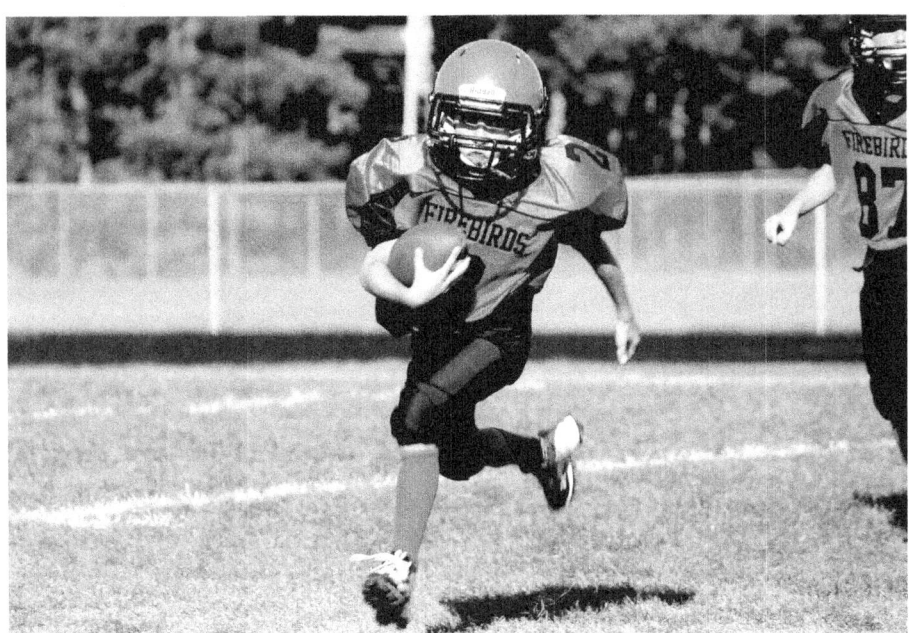

INTRODUCTION

Welcome to offensive football! Since you put down hard-earned money to purchase this book (thank you!), we imagine you have a keen interest in coaching youth football and learning more about concepts that can help your team move the ball and score points consistently. If you are hard working, creative, and detail-oriented, this experience will be a lot of fun.

What follows are diagrams and individual player assignments for 114 plays designed for tackle football players aged 8-12. They encompass not only plays that our teams have used but many sound plays run over the years by our opponents. These can serve as the basis of your team's playbook, or as the starting point for completely new plays you and your staff draw up. That is the beauty of offensive football — there are endless ways to move the ball.

Before diving in, here are some things to consider.

- We aim to enter games with 10-12 bread and butter plays, capable of being run either left or right, and 5-6 additional one-off plays with special formations or actions. This comes to roughly 30 total plays. Resist the urge add too much beyond this — you will not have the time to practice these plays sufficiently, or if you do you will likely be neglecting other important fundamentals.

- When possible, install complementary plays run from the same formation that build off each other. For instance, 26 Lead sets up 26 Bootleg, 26 Bootleg Pass, and 26 Bootleg Shovel Pass. Most players' assignments are the same or similar for each, with slight changes, so you are really getting four plays in one.

- The majority of the plays in this book are depicted with the quarterback under center. In recent years our teams have increasingly used the shotgun to great effect. Either method can be effective, and play assignments do not change dramatically. See what your kids can handle before committing to either.

- In our experience the widest possible line splits create optimum running conditions. There are certainly times when this is not the case, like when your team has a considerable size advantage on the opposition and pounding the ball behind all that beef is your best bet. But for average or undersized teams, wide splits create larger running lanes, and blocking struggles can be addressed with numbers, angles, and misdirection.

- Passing is certainly possible in youth football, but consider what your kids can do. In full equipment, even the strongest-armed child will only be able to throw the ball 20-25 yards in the air. In addition, you should not expect Joe Thomas-level pass protection from your offensive line, or a quarterback who can cycle through multiple progressions. Consider all of these variables when planning your receivers' routes, the number of receivers in each route, and the number of players you devote to pass protection.

- Whatever plays you choose to run, the installation process is critical in your players' understanding of what you are trying to accomplish. Consider using a whiteboard to draw up formations and illustrate player assignments. In the preseason we install 3-4 plays per day, running them as an 11-player unit on air before drilling skills in smaller position groups, then reconvening to run them against a scout defense. As you teach your players the offense, consider their learning styles and tailor your approach to the greatest number of kids.

- Take video of as many of your activities as possible. Game video is a must, but practice video can be just as important. Use video to analyze flaws in your play design or execution, and adjust accordingly. Or, if everything works perfectly, celebrate with your kids! Capturing and reviewing video does not need to be expensive or time consuming — no grinding the remote until 3 a.m. necessary — but can really help you teach your kids the game better and put them in position for maximum success.

- These plays are diagrammed to be run against a 5-3 defense where defensive linemen are required to line up directly across from offensive linemen. It is certainly possible to run these plays against a 4-4, 6-2, 4-3, or other fronts.

We could go on and on, but you want to get to these plays. So give them a look, and let us know what you think. Email me at scott_tappa@hotmail.com, connect on Twitter at @scotttappa, and let's help make each other better!

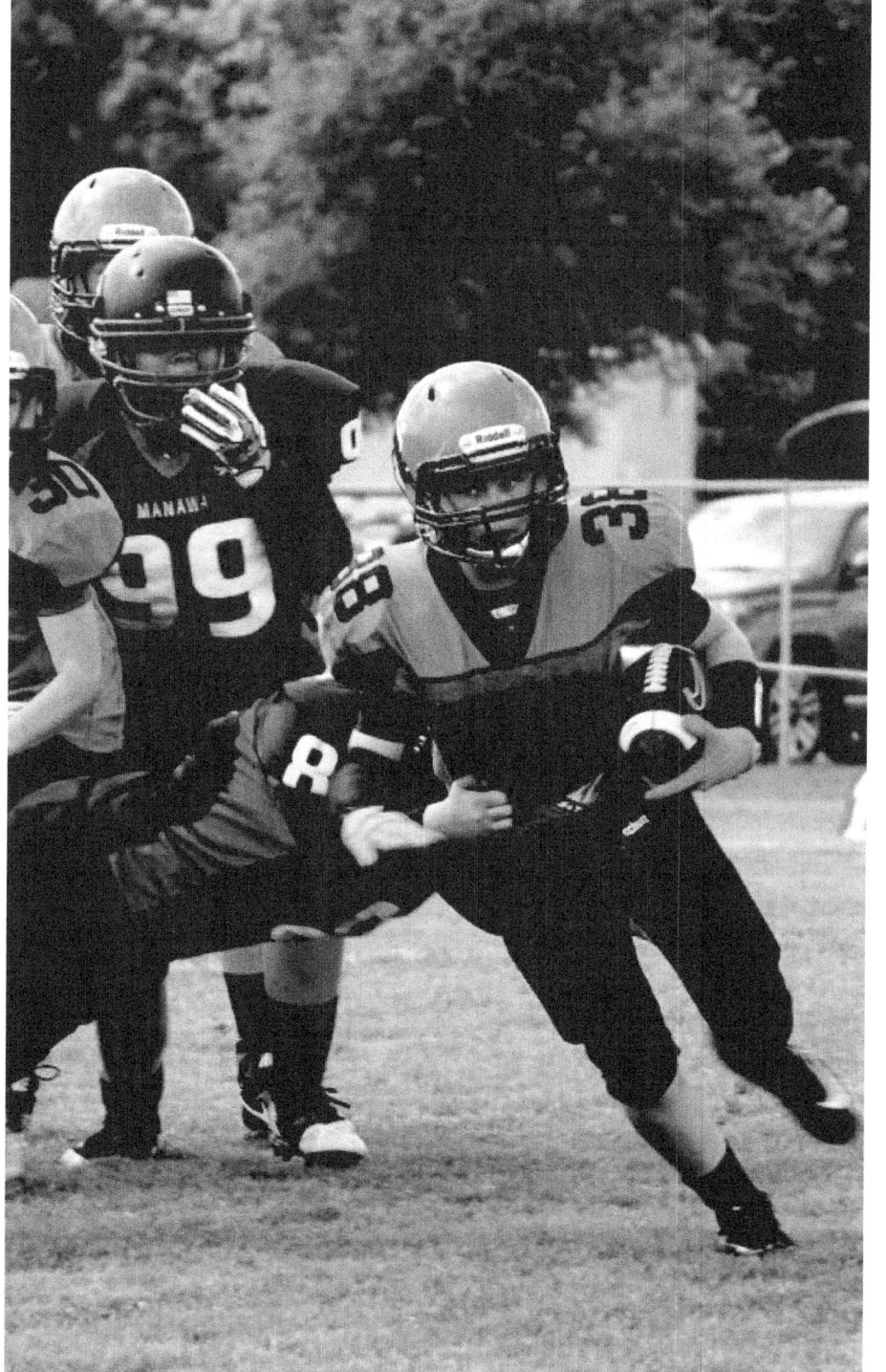

OFFENSE OVERVIEW

Positions

C – Center
G – Guard
T – Tackle
TE – Tight End
SE – Split End
TH – Thunderback
FB – Fullback
HB – Halfback
QB – Quarterback

Back/End Numbers

1 – Quarterback
2 – Halfback
3 – Fullback
4 – Thunderback/Wingback
5 – Split End
6 – Tight End

Typical Lineup

Center – On ball
Guard – Fingertip-to-fingertip split
Tackle – Fingertip-to-fingertip split
Tight End – Fingertip-to-fingertip split next to tackle
Split End – Split 5-10 yards outside tackle on line of scrimmage (normal) OR – fingertip-to-fingertip split next to tackle (tight)
Thunderback – Split 3 yards outside tight end, 2-3 yards behind line of scrimmage
Fullback – 3 yards behind quarterback
Halfback – 2 yards behind fullback
Quarterback – Under center or in shotgun

Typical Formation
Offense Positions and Holes

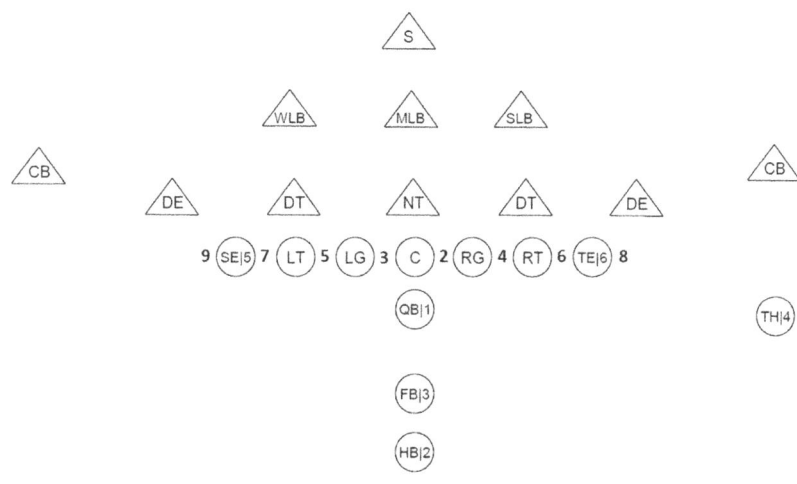

Must have seven players on line of scrimmage; split receivers must check with side referee to make sure they are properly aligned

Offensive Series

Lead Series – Fullback leads halfback through hole, setting up bootleg and bootleg pass

Pitch series – Pitch to halfback for perimeter run, setting up pitch pass and reverse

Quick series – Quarterback sneak, quick handoff to fullback, quick pass to tight ends

Keeper series – Quarterback perimeter runs, setting up reverse, pass

Rocket series – Thunderback sweep from motion, setting up halfback/fullback dive, play action pass

Twins series – Two receivers run routes to same side

Trips series – Three receivers split to same side

Empty series – Trips right, twins left or vice versa

Cadence

Down, ready, set, hut

PLAY NAMES

The plays in this book follow standard naming conventions. In all cases these elements can be altered to suit your preferences. Let's take a look at the play call Gun Right 26 Lead. The basic elements include:

Formation: Instructs offensive players where to line up. For instance, in this book Gun Right calls for the quarterback to line up in the shotgun, and the Thunderback to line up to the right side of the formation. The offense has more players to the right side of the center, hence "Gun Right." If the quarterback was under center, we would call this formation "Strong Right."

Back number: The first of the two-digit number, in this play 2, indicates which player will carry the ball. For purposes of this book, 1=quarterback, 2=halfback, 3=fullback, 4=Thunderback (or wingback), 5=split end, 6=tight end. In this play the halfback will carry the ball.

Hole number: The second of the two-digit number, in this play 6, indicates which hole the ball carrier will run through. Hole numbers to the right of center are even numbers starting at 2, while hole numbers to the left of center are odd numbers starting at 3. In this play the halfback will run through the 6 hole, which is the hole between the right tackle and tight end.

Action: The last part of the play name indicates any key actions. In this play "lead" indicates that the fullback will lead the halfback through the 6 hole, and the halfback will cut off the fullback's lead block. These actions can be as long and descriptive as you think appropriate, but we suggest keeping play names as short and simple as possible. You are not dealing with NFL players here!

LEAD SERIES

Strong Right 26 Lead

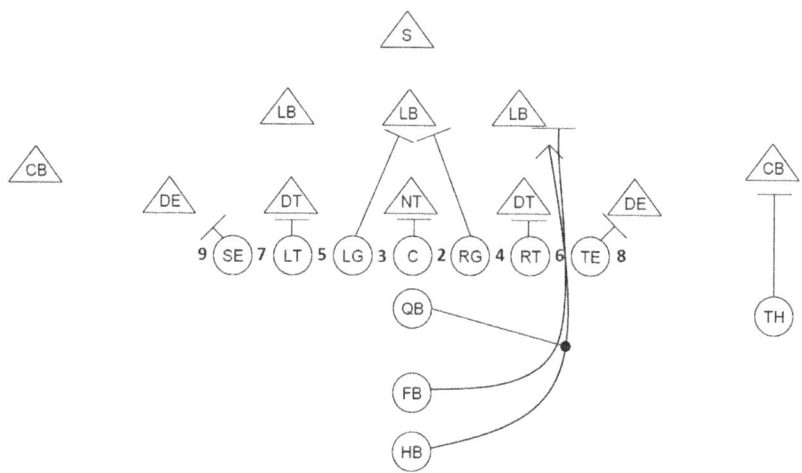

SE: Block DE, first step right foot
LT: Block DT, first step right foot
LG: Chip NT with right arm, climb to MLB
C: Block NT
RG: Chip NT with left arm, climb to MLB
RT: Block DT, first step right foot
TE: Block DE, first step left foot
TH: Block CB or double team DE with TE
QB: First step right foot, meet HB between 4 and 6 holes for handoff, hand off with left hand, carry out bootleg fake after handing off
FB: First step right foot, lead HB through 6 hole, pick up first unblocked defender, likely OLB
HB: First step right foot, meet QB for handoff between and 6 holes, two arms protecting ball through 6 hole, cut off FB block

LEAD SERIES

Strong Right 26 Power

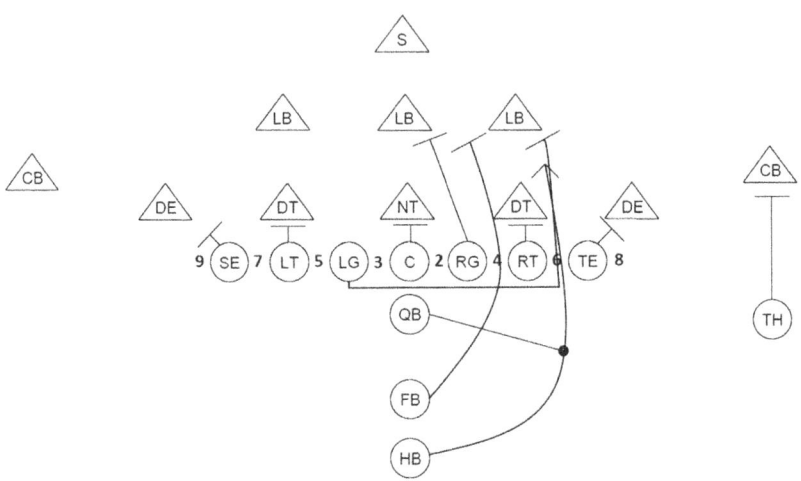

SE: Block DE, first step right foot

LT: Block DT, first step right foot

LG: Bucket step with right foot, turn shoulders toward sideline and pull, square up and lead through 6 hole, pick up first unblocked defender, likely OLB

C: Block NT

RG: Chip NT with left arm, climb to MLB

RT: Block DT, first step right foot

TE: Block DE, first step left foot

TH: Block CB or double team DE with TE

QB: First step right foot, meet HB between 4 and 6 holes for handoff, hand off with left hand, carry out bootleg fake after handing off

FB: First step right foot, move through 4 hole, block MLB

HB: First step right foot, meet QB for handoff between 4 and 6 holes, two arms protecting ball through 6 hole, cut off LG block

LEAD SERIES

Strong Left 26 Bootleg

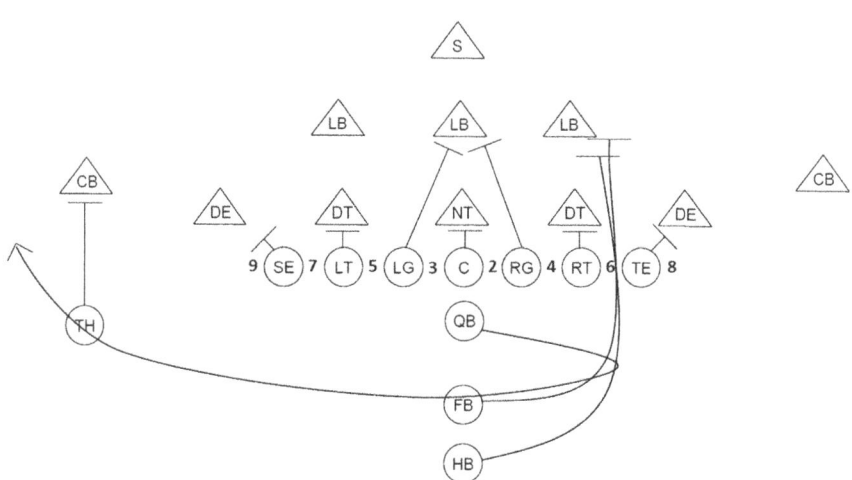

SE: Block DE, first step right foot
LT: Block DT, first step right foot
LG: Chip NT with right arm, climb to MLB
C: Block NT
RG: Chip NT with left arm, climb to MLB
RT: Block DT, first step right foot
TE: Block DE, first step left foot
TH: Block CB or double team DE with TE
QB: First step right foot, meet HB between 4 and 6 holes for handoff, fake handoff with left hand, make tight turn (no deeper than 3 yards), get outside to 9 hole
FB: First step right foot, lead HB through 6 hole, pick up first unblocked defender, likely OLB
HB: First step right foot, meet QB between 4 and 6 holes, carry out fake handoff through 6 hole

LEAD SERIES

Strong Left 26 Bootleg Pass

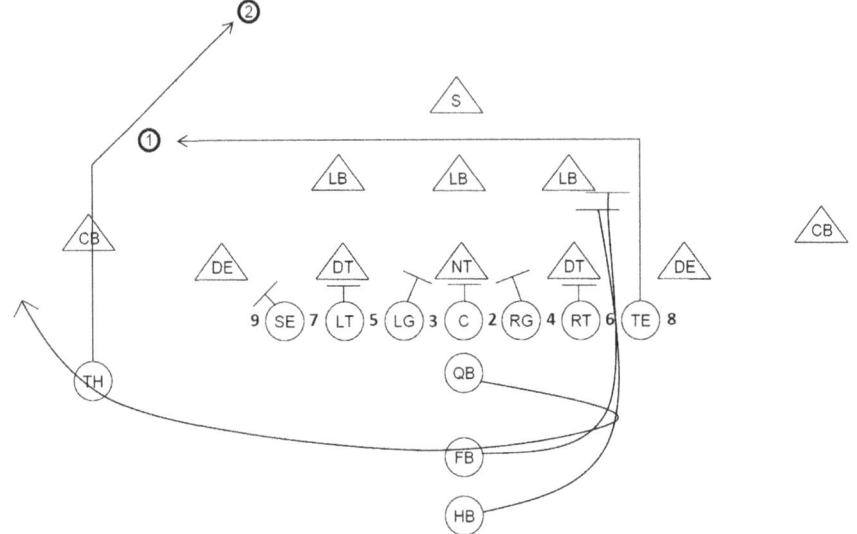

Note: SE through RT can not block further than 3 yards downfield
SE: Block DE, first step right foot
LT: Block DT, first step right foot
LG: Triple team NT, prepare to pick up blitz if necessary
C: Block NT
RG: Triple team NT, prepare to pick up blitz if necessary
RT: Block DT, first step right foot
TE: Chip DE, then release to crossing route behind linebackers, 5 yards, planting with right foot for 90-degree cut
TH: Run 5-yard post, planting with left foot for 45-degree cut
QB: First step right foot, meet HB between 4 and 6 holes for handoff, fake handoff with left hand, make tight turn (no deeper than 3 yards), get outside to 9 hole, planting and throwing to open receiver (run option if neither receiver is open)
FB: First step right foot, lead HB through 6 hole, pick up first unblocked defender
HB: First step right foot, meet QB between 4 and 6 holes, carry out fake handoff

LEAD SERIES

Gun Left 26 Bootleg Shovel Pass

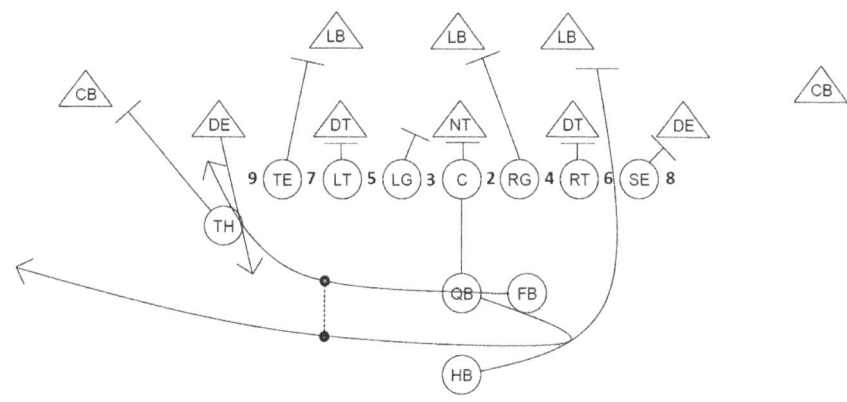

Note: SE through RT can not block further than 3 yards downfield
SE: Block DE, first step left foot
LT: Block DT, first step left foot
LG: Double team NT with C
C: Block NT
RG: Chip on NT with left arm before climbing to MLB
RT: Block DT, first step left foot
TE: Chip on DT with right arm before climbing to OLB
TH: Block CB
QB: First step right foot, meet HB between 4 and 6 holes for handoff, fake handoff with left hand, make tight turn (no deeper than 3 yards), throw shovel pass to FB when he is between playside DE and line of scrimmage, if DE stays home run with ball with FB as lead blocker
FB: Jab step right with right foot, faking block to 6 hole, turn shoulders toward left sideline and run parallel down line, aiming to fit between line of scrimmage and playside DE, look for shovel pass from QB
HB: First step right foot, meet QB between 4 and 6 holes, carry out fake handoff

LEAD SERIES

Pro Right 34 Crossbuck

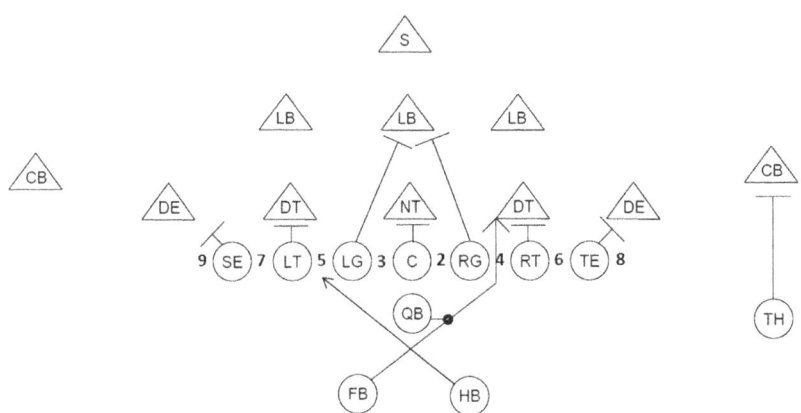

SE: Block DE, first step right foot
LT: Block DT, first step right foot
LG: Chip NT with right arm, climb to MLB
C: Block NT
RG: Chip NT with left arm, climb to MLB or OLB, depending on how they flow
RT: Block DT, first step left foot
TE: Block DE, first step left foot
TH: Block CB or double team DE with TE
QB: Pivot left after receiving snap, faking handoff to HB heading for 5 hole, continue pivot and hand off to FB heading for 4 hole
FB: Exaggerated jab step with left foot, throwing up arms for emphasis, faking lead block through 5 hole, then cutting back off left foot, receiving handoff from QB and running through 4 hole
HB: First step left foot, meet QB behind 3 hole, carry out fake handoff

LEAD SERIES

Pro Right 36 Lead

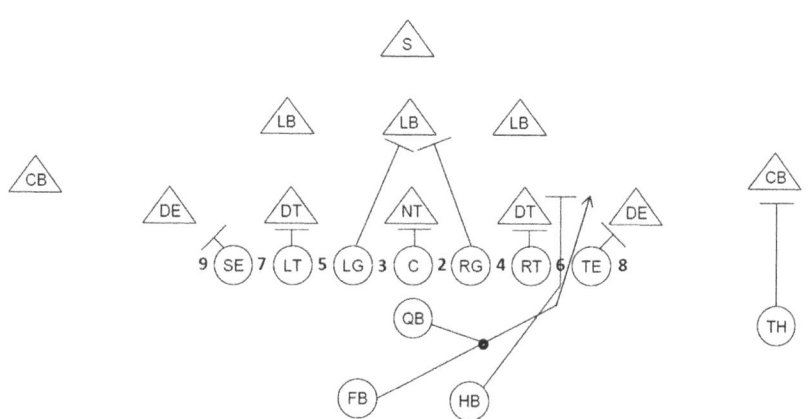

SE: Block DE, first step right foot
LT: Block DT, first step right foot
LG: Chip NT with right arm, climb to MLB
C: Block NT
RG: Chip NT with left arm, climb to MLB
RT: Block DT, first step right foot
TE: Block DE, first step left foot
TH: Block CB or double team DE with TE
QB: First step right foot, meet FB behind 4 hole for handoff, hand off with left hand, carry out bootleg fake after handing off
FB: First step right foot, meet QB for handoff behind 4 hole, two arms protecting ball through hole, cut off HB block
HB: First step right foot, lead FB through 6 hole, pick up first unblocked defender, likely OLB

LEAD SERIES

Pro Right 38 Lead

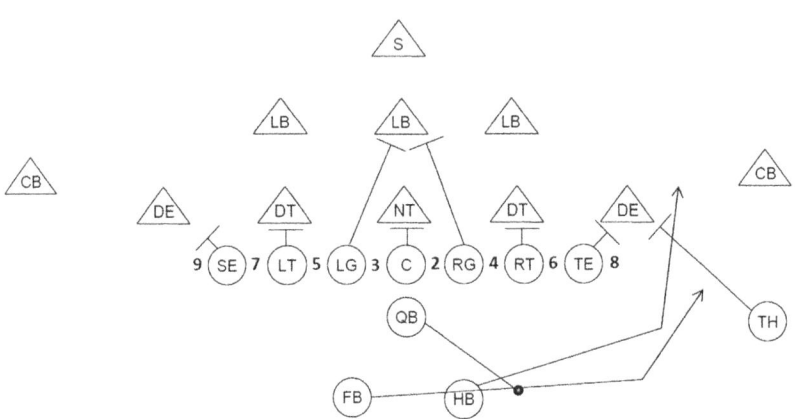

SE: Block DE, first step right foot

LT: Block DT, first step right foot

LG: Chip NT with right arm, climb to MLB

C: Block NT

RG: Chip NT with left arm, climb to MLB

RT: Block DT, first step right foot

TE: Block DE, first step left foot

TH: Double team DE with TE

QB: First step right foot, meet FB behind 4 hole for handoff, hand off with left hand, carry out bootleg fake after handing off

FB: First step right foot, meet QB for handoff behind 4 hole, two arms protecting ball through hole, follow HB outside around end, cut off HB block

HB: First step right foot, lead FB through around end, pick up first unblocked defender, likely OLB or CB

LEAD SERIES

Pro Right 36 Play Action

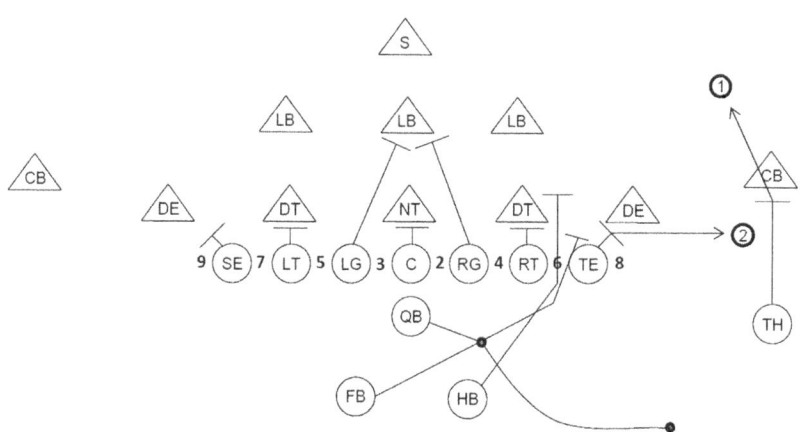

Note: SE through RT can not block further than 3 yards downfield
SE: Block DE, first step right foot
LT: Block DT, first step right foot
LG: Triple team NT, prepare to pick up blitz if necessary
C: Block NT
RG: Triple team NT, prepare to pick up blitz if necessary
RT: Block DT, first step right foot
TE: Chip DE, first step left foot, then release into flat
TH: Chip CB as if run blocking, then release to post route, cutting off right foot
QB: First step right foot, meet FB behind 4 hole, fake handoff, then roll outside pocket and throw to open receiver
FB: First step right foot, meet QB behind 4 hole, carry out fake handoff through 6 hole
HB: First step right foot, lead FB through 6 hole, pick up first unblocked defender, likely OLB

LEAD SERIES

Pro Left 25 Crossbuck

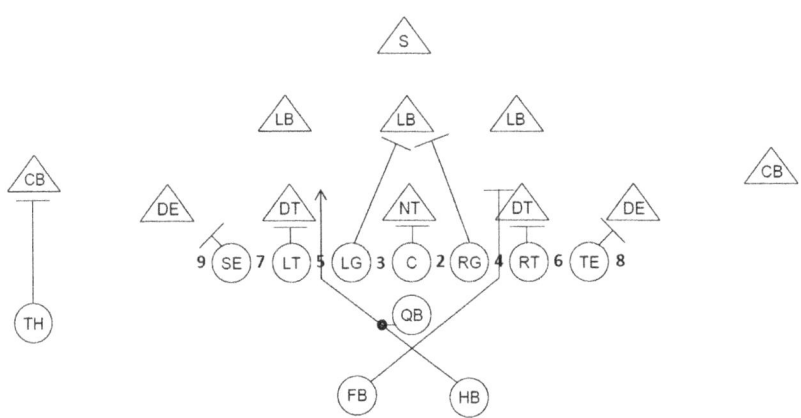

SE: Block DE, first step right foot
LT: Block DT, first step right foot
LG: Chip NT with right arm, climb to MLB or OLB, depending on how they flow
C: Block NT
RG: Chip NT with left arm, climb to MLB
RT: Block DT, first step left foot
TE: Block DE, first step left foot
TH: Block CB or double team DE with TE
QB: Pivot right after receiving snap, faking handoff to FB heading for 4 hole, continue pivot and hand off to HB heading for 5 hole
FB: First step right foot, meet QB behind 2 hole, carry out fake handoff
HB: Exaggerated jab step with right foot, throwing up arms for emphasis, faking lead block through 4 hole, then cutting back off right foot, receiving handoff from QB and running through 5 hole

LEAD SERIES

Pro Left 27 Lead

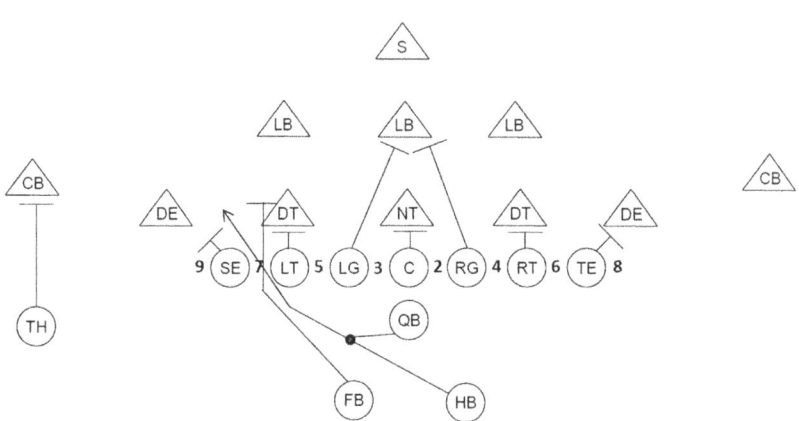

SE: Block DE, first step right foot
LT: Block DT, first step left foot
LG: Chip NT with right arm, climb to MLB
C: Block NT
RG: Chip NT with left arm, climb to MLB
RT: Block DT, first step left foot
TE: Block DE, first step left foot
TH: Block CB or double team DE with SE
QB: First step left foot, meet HB behind 5 hole for handoff, hand off with right hand, carry out bootleg fake after handing off
FB: First step left foot, lead HB through 7 hole, pick up first unblocked defender, likely OLB
HB: First step left foot, meet QB for handoff behind 5 hole, two arms protecting ball through hole, cut off FB block

LEAD SERIES

Pro Left 29 Lead

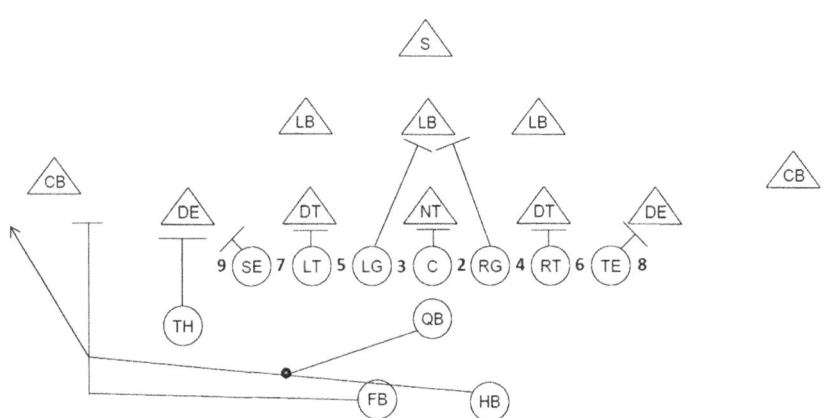

SE: Block DE, first step right foot
LT: Block DT, first step left foot
LG: Chip NT with right arm, climb to MLB
C: Block NT
RG: Chip NT with left arm, climb to MLB
RT: Block DT, first step left foot
TE: Block DE, first step left foot
TH: Double team DE with SE
QB: First step left foot, meet HB behind 7 hole for handoff, hand off with right hand, carry out bootleg fake after handing off
FB: First step left foot, lead HB around end, pick up first unblocked defender, likely CB or OLB
HB: First step left foot, meet QB for handoff behind 7 hole, follow FB outside around end, cut off FB block

LEAD SERIES

Strong Left 27 Lead

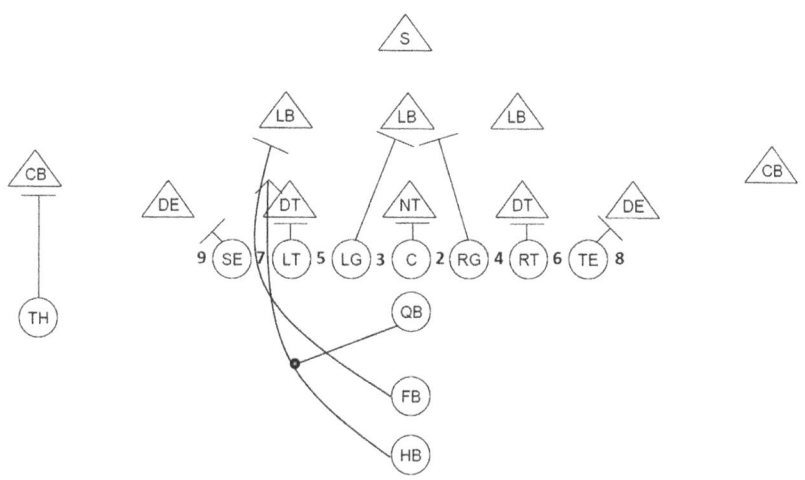

SE: Block DE, first step right foot
LT: Block DT, first step left foot
LG: Chip NT with right arm, climb to MLB
C: Block NT
RG: Chip NT with left arm, climb to MLB
RT: Block DT, first step left foot
TE: Block DE, first step left foot
TH: Block CB or double team DE with SE
QB: First step left foot, meet HB between 5 and 7 holes for handoff, hand off with right hand, carry out bootleg fake after handing off
FB: First step left foot, lead HB through 7 hole, pick up first unblocked defender, likely OLB
HB: First step left foot, meet QB for handoff between 5 and 7 holes, two arms protecting ball through hole, cut off FB block

LEAD SERIES

Strong Left 27 Power

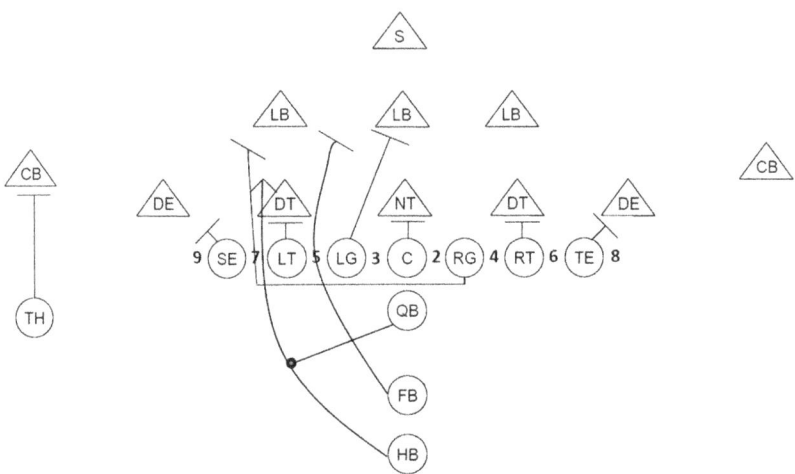

SE: Block DE, first step right foot
LT: Block DT, first step left foot
LG: Chip NT with right arm, climb to MLB
C: Block NT
RG: Bucket step with left foot, turn shoulders toward sideline and pull, square up and lead through 7 hole, pick up first unblocked defender, likely OLB
RT: Block DT, first step left foot
TE: Block DE, first step left foot
TH: Block CB or double team DE with TE
QB: First step left foot, meet HB between 5 and 7 holes for handoff, hand off with right hand, carry out bootleg fake after handing off
FB: First step left foot, move through 5 hole, block MLB
HB: First step left foot, meet QB for handoff between 5 and 7 holes, two arms protecting ball through hole, cut off RG block

LEAD SERIES

Strong Right 27 Bootleg

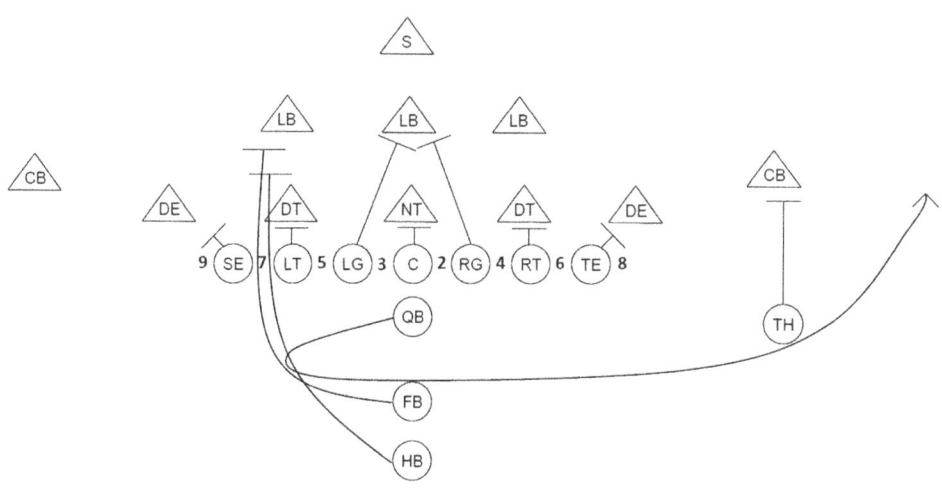

SE: Block DE, first step right foot
LT: Block DT, first step left foot
LG: Chip NT with right arm, climb to MLB
C: Block NT
RG: Chip NT with left arm, climb to MLB
RT: Block DT, first step right foot
TE: Block DE, first step left foot
TH: Block CB or double team DE with TE
QB: First step left foot, meet HB between 5 and 7 holes for handoff, fake handoff with right hand, make tight turn (no deeper than 3 yards), get outside to 8 hole, reading TE and TH blocks
FB: First step left foot, lead HB through 7 hole, pick up first unblocked defender, likely OLB
HB: First step left foot, meet QB between 5 and 7 holes, carry out fake handoff

LEAD SERIES

Strong Right 27 Bootleg Pass

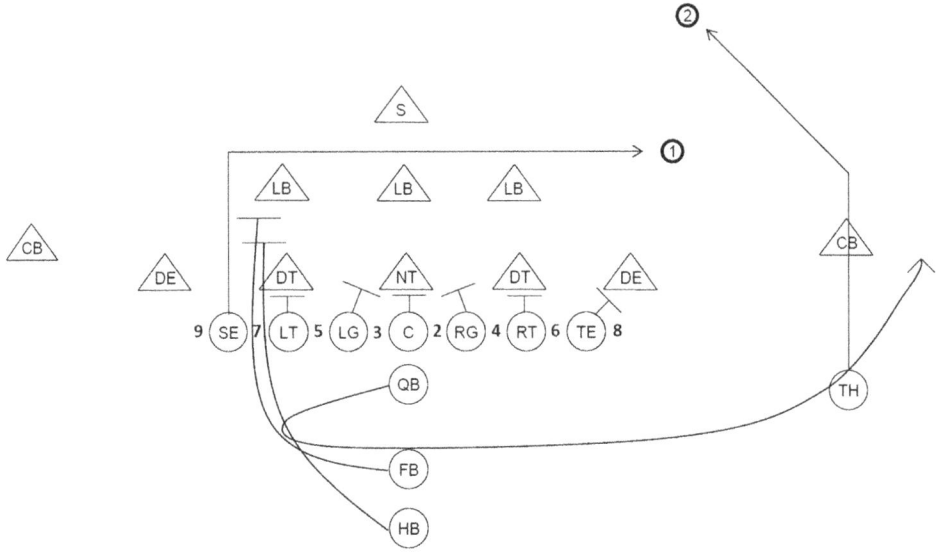

Note: LT through TE can not block further than 3 yards downfield

SE: Chip DE, then release to crossing route behind linebackers, 5 yards, planting with left foot for 90-degree cut

LT: Block DT, first step right foot

LG: Triple team NT, prepare to pick up blitz if necessary

C: Block NT

RG: Triple team NT, prepare to pick up blitz if necessary

RT: Block DT, first step right foot

TE: Block DE, first step right foot

TH: Run 5-yard post route, planting with right foot for 45-degree cut

QB: First step left foot, meet HB between 5 and 7 holes for handoff, fake handoff with right hand, make tight turn (no deeper than 3 yards), get outside to 8 hole, planting and throwing to open receiver (run option if neither receiver is open)

FB: First step left foot, lead HB through 7 hole, pick up first unblocked defender, likely OLB

HB: First step left foot, meet QB between 5 and 7 holes, carry out fake handoff

LEAD SERIES

Gun Right 27 Bootleg Screen

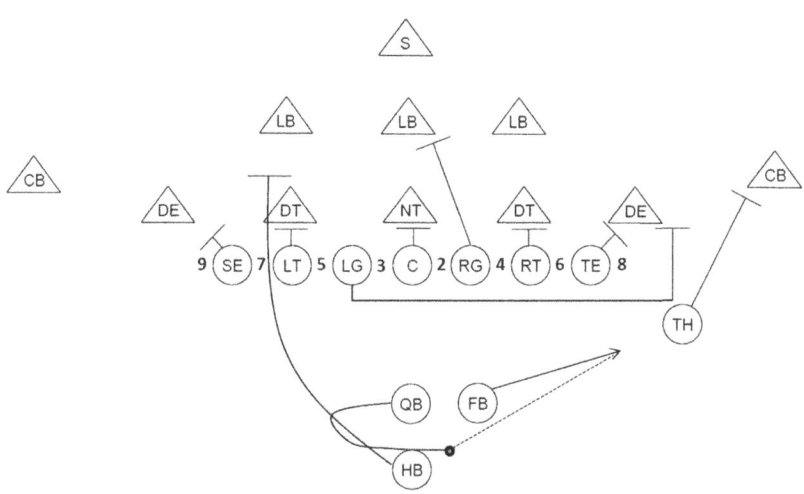

SE: Block DE, first step right foot

LT: Block DT, first step right foot

LG: Bucket step with right foot, turn shoulders toward sideline and pull, square up and lead around, pick up first unblocked defender, likely OLB

C: Block NT

RG: Chip NT with left arm before climbing to MLB

RT: Block DT, first step right foot

TE: Block DE, first step right foot

TH: Block CB

QB: First step left foot, meet HB between 5 and 7 holes for handoff, fake handoff with right hand, make tight turn, throw to FB

FB: Jab step left with left foot, faking block to 7 hole, then releasing to right flat, looking over right shoulder for pass, following lead block of LG

HB: First step left foot, meet QB between 5 and 7 holes, carry out fake handoff

LEAD SERIES

Gun Right 27 Bootleg Shovel Pass

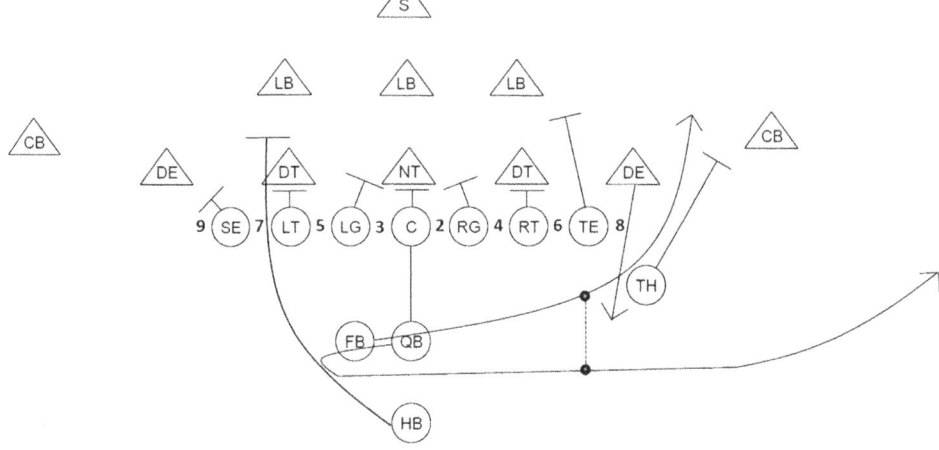

Note: SE through RT can not block further than 3 yards downfield

SE: Block DE, first step right foot

LT: Block DT, first step right foot

LG: Triple team NT with C

C: Block NT

RG: Triple team NT with C

RT: Block DT, first step right foot

TE: Chip on DT with left arm before climbing to OLB

TH: Block CB

QB: First step left foot, meet HB between 5 and 7 holes, fake handoff, make tight turn (no deeper than 3 yards), throw shovel pass to FB between playside DE and line of scrimmage, if DE stays home run with ball with FB as lead blocker

FB: Jab step left with left foot, faking block to 7 hole, turn shoulders toward right sideline and run parallel down line, aiming to fit between line of scrimmage and playside DE, look for shovel pass from QB

HB: First step left foot, meet QB between 5 and 7 holes, carry out fake handoff

LEAD SERIES

Pro Left 27 Play Action

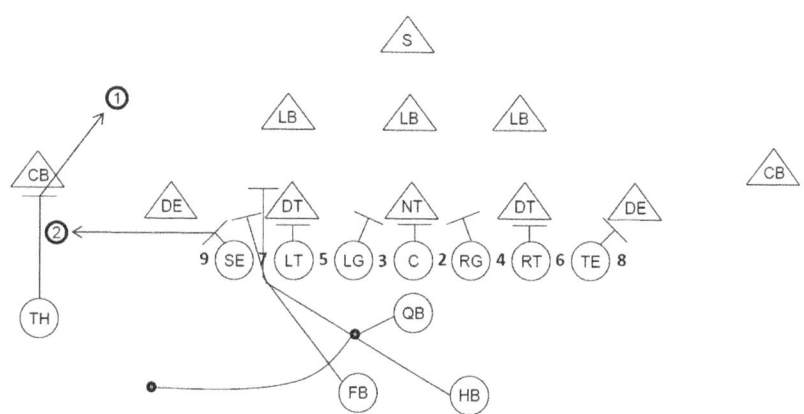

Note: LT through TE can not block further than 3 yards downfield

SE: Chips DE, first step right foot, then release into left flat, turning head over left shoulder

LT: Block DT, first step left foot

LG: Triple team NT with C

C: Block NT

RG: Triple team NT with C

RT: Block DT, first step left foot

TE: Block DE, first step left foot

TH: Stalk block CB, then release at 5 yards to post

QB: First step left, meet HB behind 5 hole, fake handoff, roll left, set feet and throw to open receiver

FB: First step left, lead block through 7 hole

HB: First step left, meet QB behind 5 hole, carry out fake handoff

LEAD SERIES

Club Right 28 Lead

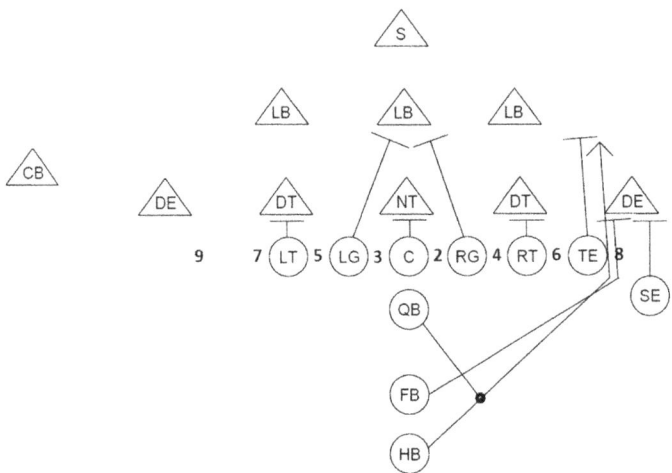

SE: Double team DE with FB, first step right foot
LT: Block DT, first step right foot
LG: Chip NT with right arm before climbing to MLB
C: Block NT
RG: Chip NT with left arm before climbing to MLB
RT: Block DT, first step right foot
TE: Block OLB, first step right foot
TH: Stalk block CB
QB: First step right foot, meet HB behind 4 hole for handoff, hand off with left hand, carry out bootleg fake after handing off
FB: First step right foot, lead HB through 8 hole, double team DE with SE
HB: First step right foot, meet QB for handoff behind 4 hole, two arms protecting ball through hole, cut off FB block

LEAD SERIES

Club Right 28 Play Action

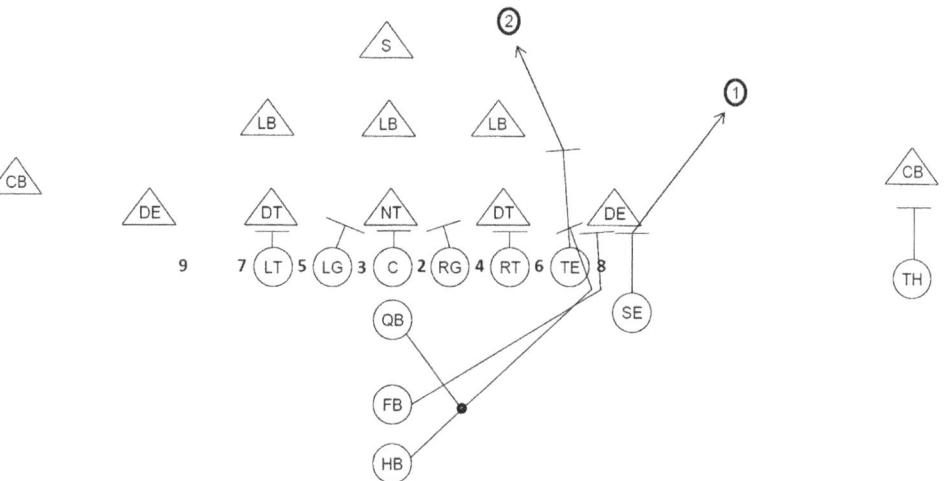

SE: First step right, chip DE, plant left foot and run corner route
LT: Block DT, first step right foot
LG: Triple team NT with C
C: Block NT
RG: Triple team NT with C
RT: Block DT, first step right foot
TE: First step right foot, faking blocking path to OLB before planting right foot and running post at 5 yards
TH: Stalk block CB
QB: First step right foot, meet HB behind 4 hole for handoff, fake hand off with left hand, take 2-3 additional steps before setting feet, passing to open receiver
FB: First step right foot, lead HB through 8 hole, block DE
HB: First step right foot, meet QB for handoff behind 4 hole, carry out fake handoff

LEAD SERIES

Club Left 29 Lead

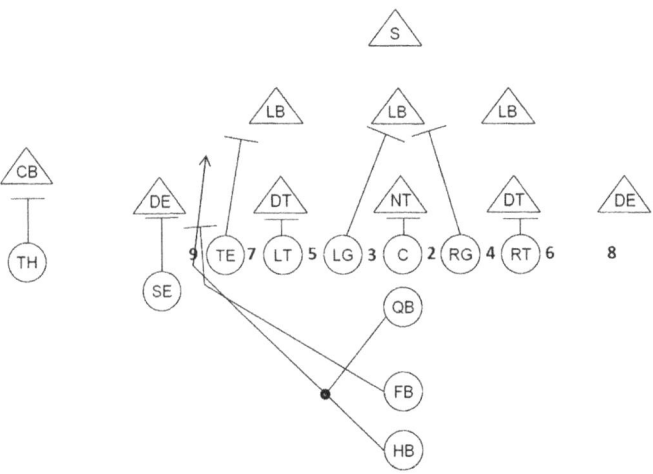

SE: Double team DE with FB, first step left foot

LT: Block DT, first step left foot

LG: Chip NT with right arm before climbing to MLB

C: Block NT

RG: Chip NT with left arm before climbing to MLB

RT: Block DT, first step left foot

TE: Block OLB, first step left foot

TH: Stalk block CB

QB: First step left foot, meet HB behind 5 hole for handoff, hand off with right hand, carry out bootleg fake after handing off

FB: First step left foot, lead HB through 9 hole, double team DE with SE

HB: First step left foot, meet QB for handoff behind 5 hole, two arms protecting ball through hole, cut off FB block

LEAD SERIES

Club Left 29 Play Action

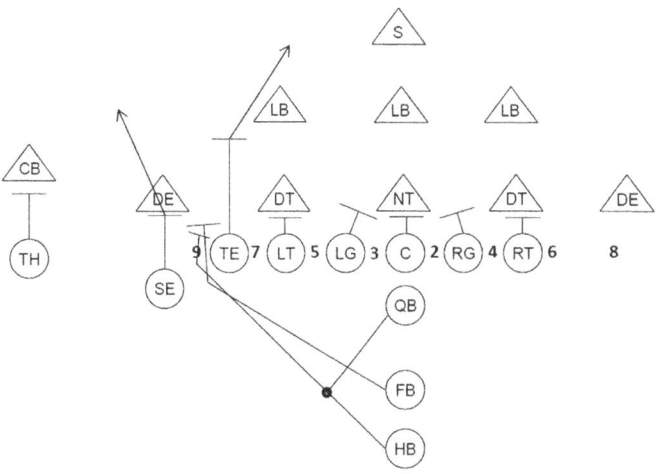

SE: First step left, chip DE, plant right foot and run corner route

LT: Block DT, first step left foot

LG: Triple team NT with C

C: Block NT

RG: Triple team NT with C

RT: Block DT, first step left foot

TE: First step left foot, faking blocking path to OLB before planting left foot and running post at 5 yards

TH: Stalk block CB

QB: First step left foot, meet HB behind 5 hole for handoff, fake hand off with right hand, take 2-3 additional steps before setting feet, passing to open receiver

FB: First step left foot, lead HB through 9 hole, block DE

HB: First step left foot, meet QB for handoff behind 5 hole, carry out fake handoff

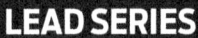

Steamroller Right 22 Lead

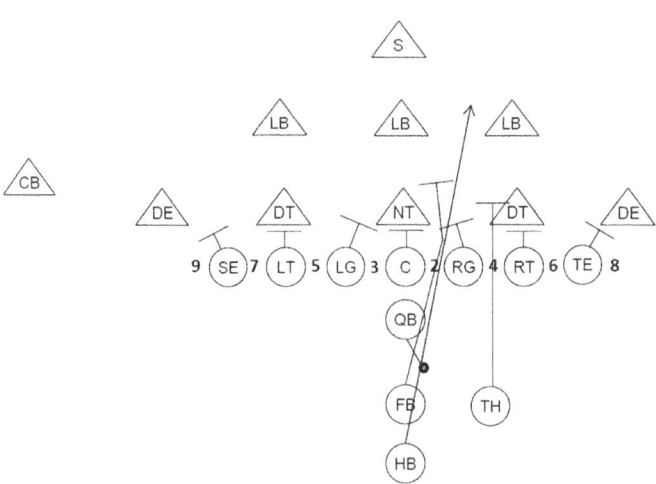

SE: Block DE, first step right foot
LT: Block DT, first step right foot
LG: Triple team NT with C
C: Block NT
RG: Triple team NT with C
RT: Block DT, first step left foot
TE: Block DE, first step left foot
TH: First step right foot, lead through 4 hole, pick up first unblocked defender, likely OLB
QB: First step right foot, quick handoff to HB heading for 2 hole, carry out bootleg fake after handing off
FB: First step right foot, lead through 2 hole, pick up first unblocked defender, likely MLB
HB: First step right foot, meet QB for handoff behind 2 hole, two arms protecting ball through hole, cut off FB, TH blocks

LEAD SERIES

Steamroller Right 22 Play Action

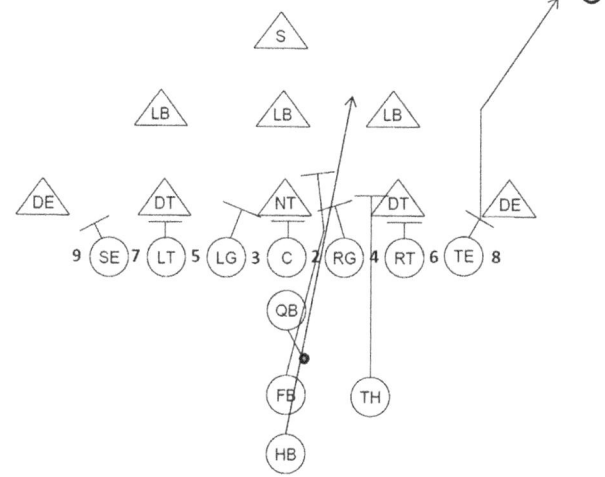

SE: Block DE, first step right foot
LT: Block DT, first step right foot
LG: Triple team NT with C
C: Block NT
RG: Triple team NT with C
RT: Block DT, first step left foot
TE: Block DE, first step left foot, before releasing to corner route, cutting off left foot at 5 yards
TH: First step right foot, lead through 4 hole, pick up first unblocked defender, likely OLB
QB: First step right foot, fake handoff to HB heading for 2 hole, take 2-3 additional steps before setting feet, passing to open receiver
FB: First step right foot, lead through 2 hole, pick up first unblocked defender, likely MLB
HB: First step right foot, meet QB for handoff behind 2 hole, carry out fake handoff

LEAD SERIES

Steamroller Left 23 Lead

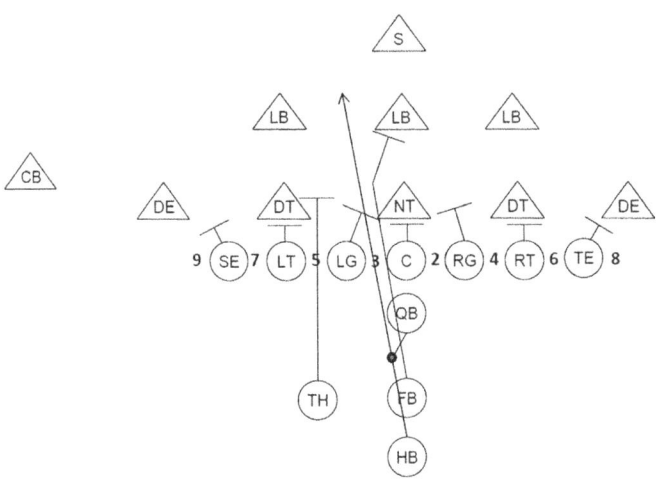

SE: Block DE, first step right foot
LT: Block DT, first step right foot
LG: Triple team NT with C
C: Block NT
RG: Triple team NT with C
RT: Block DT, first step left foot
TE: Block DE, first step left foot
TH: First step left foot, lead through 5 hole, pick up first unblocked defender, likely OLB
QB: First step left foot, quick handoff to HB heading for 3 hole, carry out bootleg fake after handing off
FB: First step left foot, lead through 3 hole, pick up first unblocked defender, likely MLB
HB: First step left foot, meet QB for handoff behind 3 hole, two arms protecting ball through hole, cut off FB, TH blocks

LEAD SERIES

Steamroller Left 23 Play Action

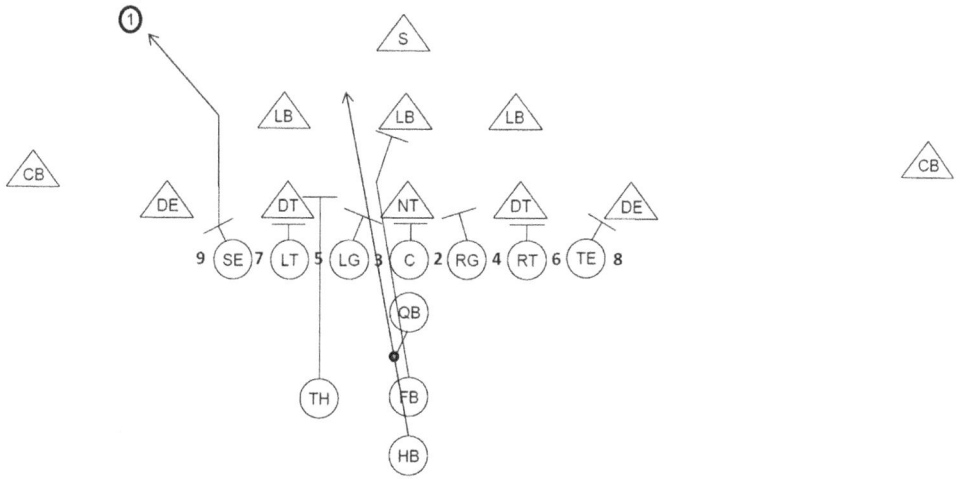

SE: Block DE, right step left foot, before releasing to corner route, cutting off right foot at 5 yards
LT: Block DT, first step right foot
LG: Triple team NT with C
C: Block NT
RG: Triple team NT with C
RT: Block DT, first step left foot
TE: Block DE, first step left foot
TH: First step left foot, lead through 5 hole, pick up first unblocked defender, likely OLB
QB: First step left foot, fake handoff to HB heading for 3 hole, take 2-3 additional steps before setting feet, passing to open receiver
FB: First step left foot, lead through 3 hole, pick up first unblocked defender, likely MLB
HB: First step left foot, meet QB for handoff behind 3 hole, carry out fake handoff

LEAD SERIES

Slots 36 Lead

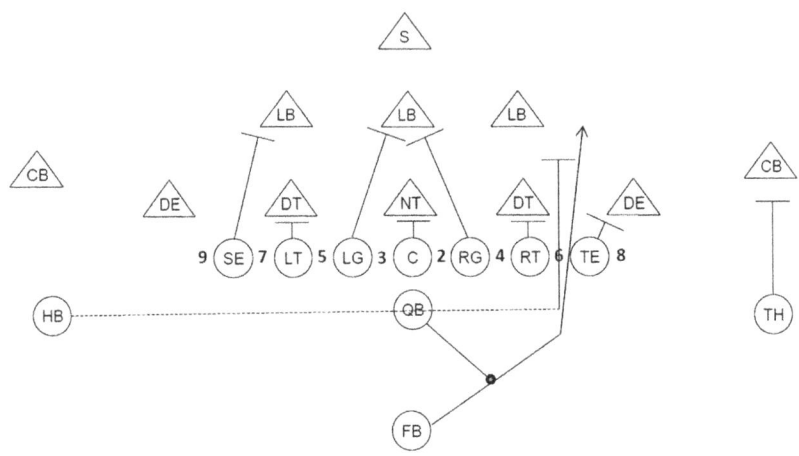

SE: Block OLB, first step left foot
LT: Block DT, first step right foot
LG: Chip NT with right arm before climbing to MLB
C: Block NT
RG: Chip NT with left arm before climbing to MLB
RT: Block DT, first step right foot
TE: Block DE, first step left foot
TH: Stalk block CB or double team DE with TE
QB: After HB passes in motion, call for snap, first step right foot, hand off to FB behind 4 hole
FB: First step right foot, aiming for 6 hole, receive hand off behind 4 hole, follow HB block through hole with two arms covering ball, cut off HB block
HB: Go in motion parallel to line of scrimmage, behind QB, on "ready," lead FB through 6 hole after snap, block OLB

LEAD SERIES

Slots 36 Play Action

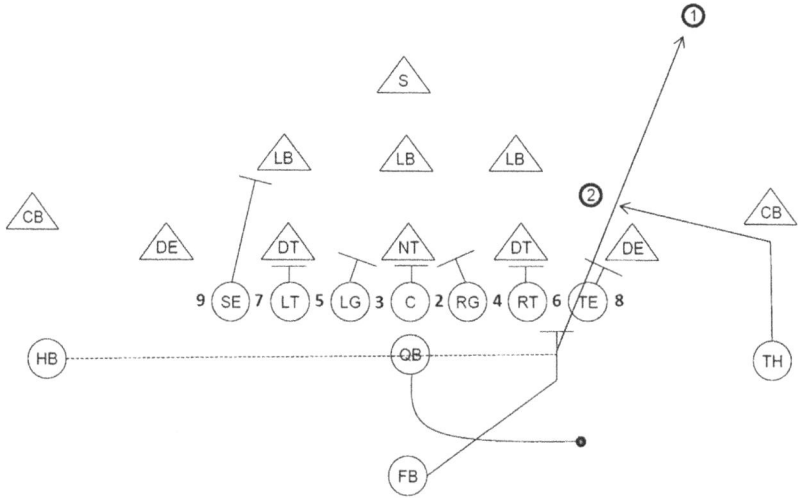

SE: Block OLB, first step left foot
LT: Block DT, first step right foot
LG: Triple team NT with C
C: Block NT
RG: Triple team NT with C
RT: Block DT, first step right foot
TE: Block DE, first step left foot
TH: Fake stalk block CB before cutting off right foot to post route
QB: After HB passes in motion, call for snap, first step right foot, fake hand off to FB behind 4 hole, take 2-3 additional steps before setting feet, passing to open receiver
FB: First step right foot, aiming for 6 hole, fake hand off behind 4 hole, carry out fake through 6 hole
HB: Go in motion parallel to line of scrimmage, behind QB, on "ready," after snap cut through 6 hole and run corner route

LEAD SERIES

Slots 37 Lead

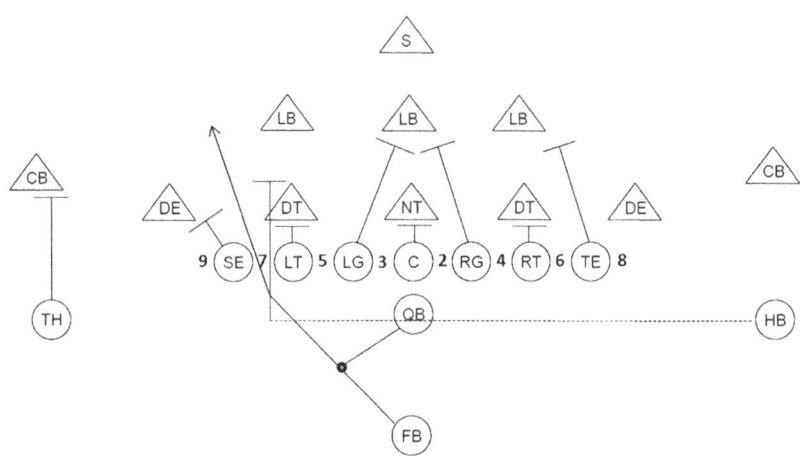

SE: Block DE, first step right foot
LT: Block DT, first step left foot
LG: Chip NT with right arm before climbing to MLB
C: Block NT
RG: Chip NT with left arm before climbing to MLB
RT: Block DT, first step left foot
TE: Block OLB, first step left foot
TH: Stalk block CB or double team DE with TE
QB: After HB passes in motion, call for snap, first step left foot, hand off to FB behind 5 hole
FB: First step left foot, aiming for 7 hole, receive hand off behind 5 hole, follow HB block through hole with two arms covering ball, cut off HB block
HB: Go in motion parallel to line of scrimmage, behind QB, on "ready," lead FB through 7 hole after snap, block OLB

LEAD SERIES

Slots 37 Play Action

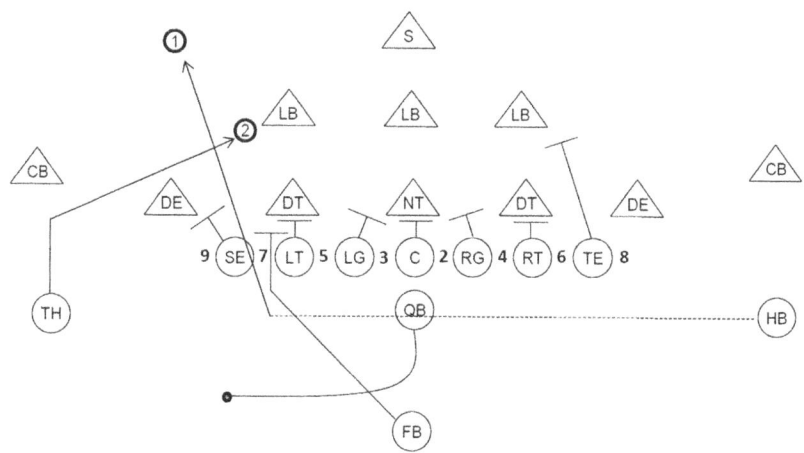

SE: Block DE, first step right foot
LT: Block DT, first step left foot
LG: Triple team NT with C
C: Block NT
RG: Triple team NT with C
RT: Block DT, first step left foot
TE: Block DE, first step left foot
TH: Fake stalk block CB before cutting off left foot to post route
QB: After HB passes in motion, call for snap, first step left foot, fake hand off to FB behind 5 hole, take 2-3 additional steps before setting feet, passing to open receiver
FB: First step left foot, aiming for 7 hole, fake hand off behind 5 hole, carry out fake through 7 hole
HB: Go in motion parallel to line of scrimmage, behind QB, on "ready," after snap cut through 7 hole and run corner route

LEAD SERIES

Wishbone 37 Counter

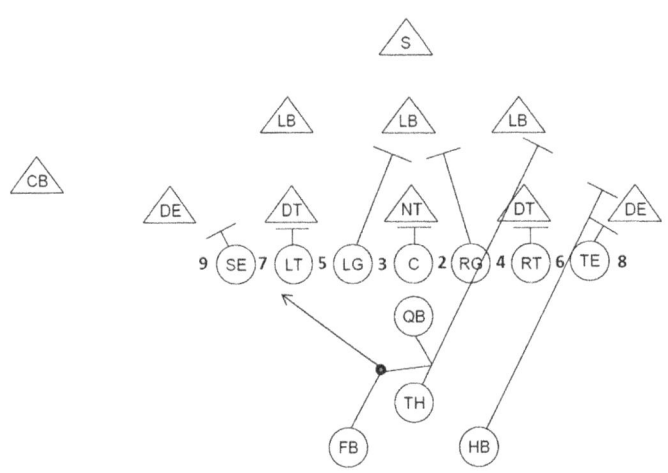

SE: Block DE, first step right foot
LT: Block DT, first step left foot
LG: Chip NT with right arm before climbing to MLB
C: Block NT
RG: Chip NT with left arm before climbing to MLB
RT: Block DT, first step left foot
TE: Block DE, first step left foot
TH: First step right foot, lead block through 4 hole
QB: First step right, fake handoff to TH behind 2 hole, continue pivot, hand off to FB behind 3 hole
FB: Jab step with right foot, faking run toward 2 hole, cut back toward 7 hole, receiving handoff from QB behind 3 hole
HB: First step right foot, lead block through 6 hole

LEAD SERIES

Wishbone 26 Counter

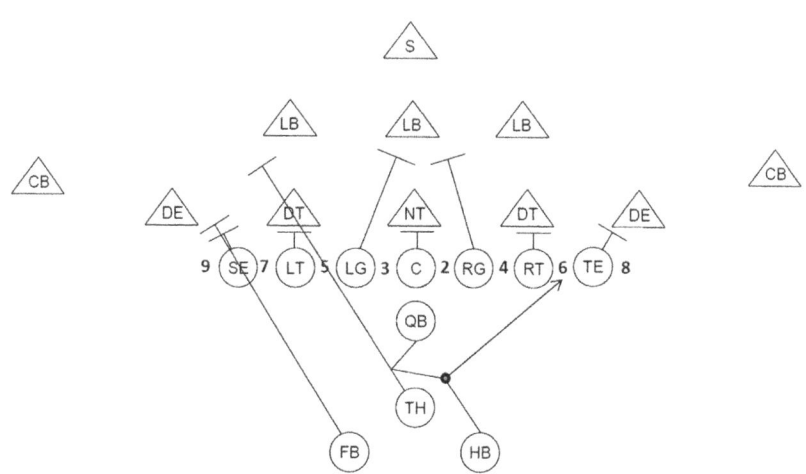

SE: Block DE, first step right foot
LT: Block DT, first step right foot
LG: Chip NT with right arm before climbing to MLB
C: Block NT
RG: Chip NT with left arm before climbing to MLB
RT: Block DT, first step right foot
TE: Block DE, first step left foot
TH: First step left foot, lead block through 5 hole
QB: First step left, fake handoff to TH behind 3 hole, continue pivot, hand off to HB behind 2 hole
FB: First step left foot, lead block through 7 hole
HB: Jab step with left foot, faking run toward 3 hole, cut back toward 6 hole, receiving handoff from QB behind 2 hole

LEAD SERIES

Machine Gun Left 19 Sweep

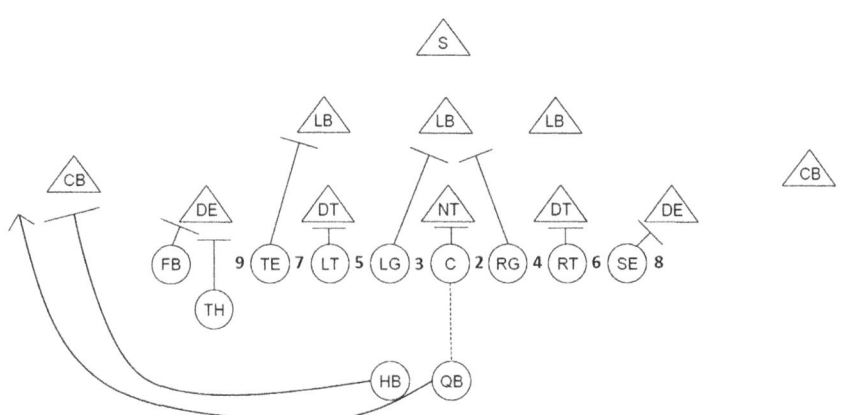

SE: Block DE, first step left foot
LT: Block DT, first step left foot
LG: Chip NT with right arm before climbing to MLB
C: Block NT
RG: Chip NT with left arm before climbing to MLB
RT: Block DT, first step left foot
TE: Block OLB, first step left foot
TH: Double team DE with FB, first step right foot
QB: Take snap and follow HB lead block around end
FB: Double team DE with TH, first step left foot
HB: Lead QB around end, picking up first unblocked defender, likely CB

LEAD SERIES

Machine Gun Left 29 Lead

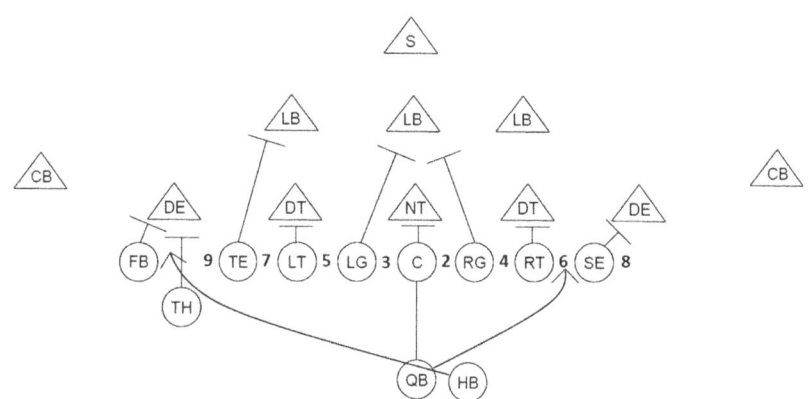

SE: Block DE, first step left foot
LT: Block DT, first step left foot
LG: Chip NT with right arm before climbing to MLB
C: Block NT
RG: Chip NT with left arm before climbing to MLB
RT: Block DT, first step left foot
TE: Block OLB, first step left foot
TH: Double team DE with FB, first step right foot
QB: Take snap and hand off to HB, then carry out fake run to 6 hole
FB: Double team DE with TH, first step left foot
HB: First step left foot, receive handoff from QB and run to 9 hole

PITCH SERIES

Strong Right 28 Pitch

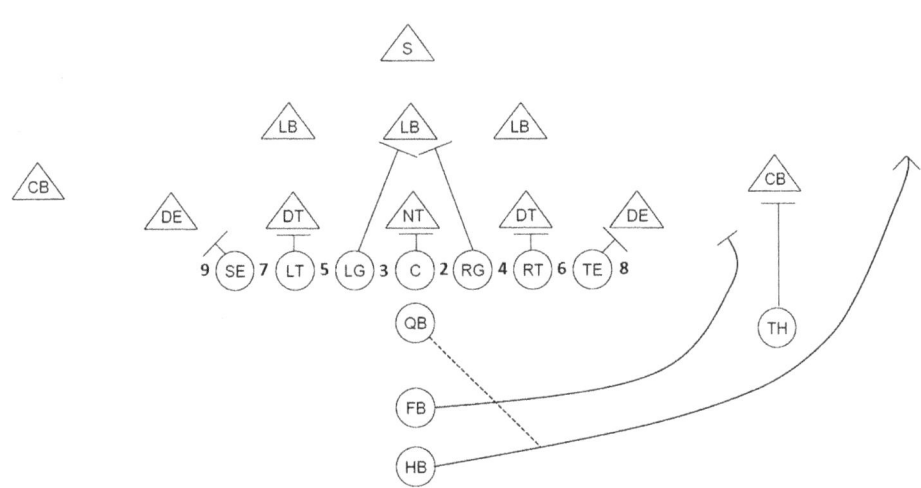

SE: Block DE, first step right foot
LT: Block DT, first step right foot
LG: Chip NT with right arm, work to MLB
C: Block NT
RG: Chip NT with left arm, work to MLB
RT: Block DT, first step right foot
TE: Block DE, first step right foot
TH: Stalk block CB or double team DE with TE
QB: Receive snap, reverse pivot, make eye contact with HB, lead HB by two steps with pitch
FB: First step right, lead HB around end, picking up first unblocked defender, likely OLB or CB
HB: First step right, get horizontal separation from QB, watch pitch into hands, follow FB lead around end

PITCH SERIES

Strong Right 28 Pitch Pass

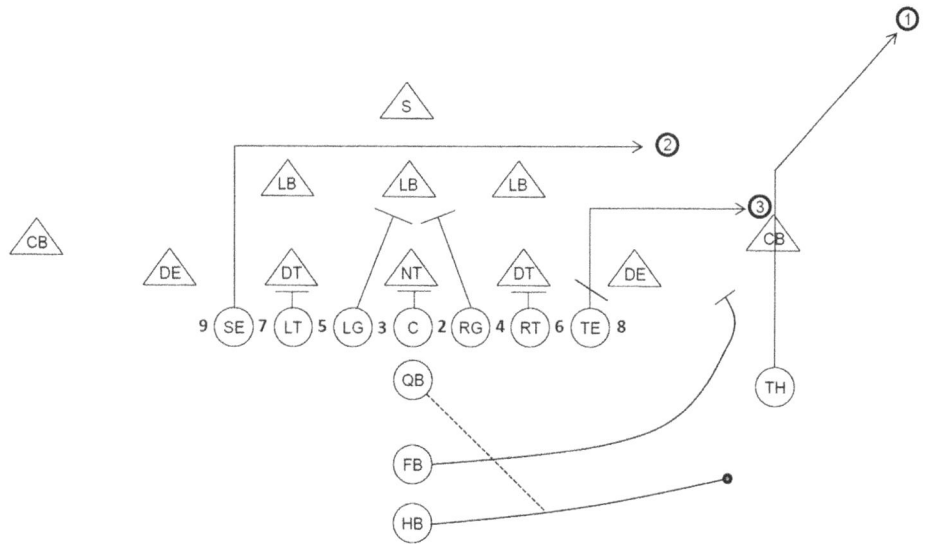

SE: Block DE, then release to crossing route behind linebackers
LT: Block DT, first step right foot
LG: Chip NT with right arm, work to MLB
C: Block NT
RG: Chip NT with left arm, work to MLB
RT: Block DT, first step right foot
TE: Block DE, then release to 3-yard out route
TH: Stalk block CB, then release to 5-yard corner route
QB: Receive snap, reverse pivot, make eye contact with HB, lead HB by two steps with pitch
FB: First step right, lead HB around end, picking up first unblocked defender, likely DE
HB: First step right, get horizontal separation from QB, watch pitch into hands, tuck ball as if running 28, then throw to open receiver

PITCH SERIES

Strong Left 29 Pitch Reverse

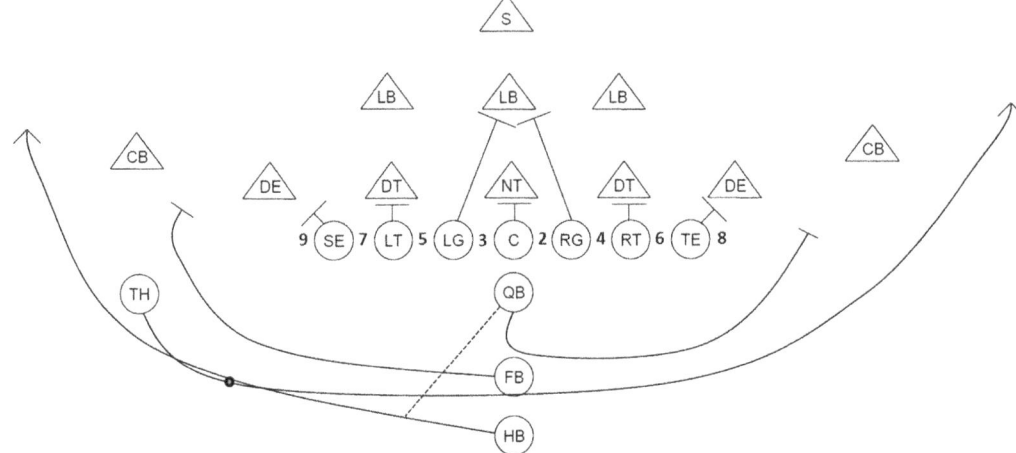

SE: Block DE, first step right foot
LT: Block DT, first step right foot
LG: Chip NT with right arm, work to MLB
C: Block NT
RG: Chip NT with left arm, work to MLB
RT: Block DT, first step right foot
TE: Block DE, first step right foot
TH: First step right foot, orbit path running opposite direction of FB and HB, receive handoff from HB, follow lead block of QB around right end
QB: Receive snap, reverse pivot, make eye contact with HB, lead HB by two steps with pitch, then lead TH around right end
FB: First step left, lead HB around end, picking up first unblocked defender, likely OLB or CB
HB: First step left, get horizontal separation from QB, watch pitch into hands, after securing ball hand off to TH with inside hand, carry out fake around left end

PITCH SERIES

Strong Left 29 Pitch

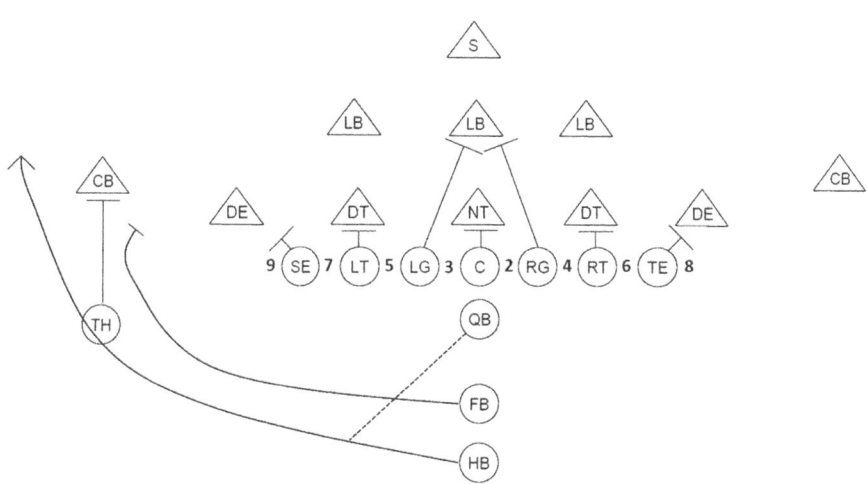

SE: Block DE, first step left foot
LT: Block DT, first step left foot
LG: Chip NT with right arm, work to MLB
C: Block NT
RG: Chip NT with left arm, work to MLB
RT: Block DT, first step left foot
TE: Block DE, first step left foot
TH: Stalk block CB or double team DE with TE
QB: Receive snap, reverse pivot, make eye contact with HB, lead HB by two steps with pitch
FB: First step left, lead HB around end, picking up first unblocked defender, likely OLB or CB
HB: First step left, get horizontal separation from QB, watch pitch into hands, follow FB lead around end

PITCH SERIES

Strong Left 29 Pitch Pass

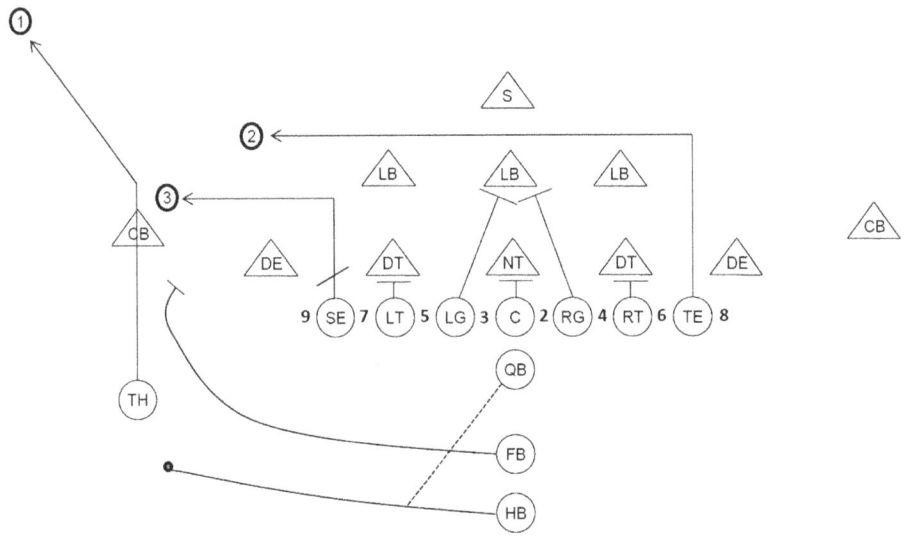

SE: Block DE, then release to 3-yard out
LT: Block DT, first step left foot
LG: Chip NT with right arm, work to MLB
C: Block NT
RG: Chip NT with left arm, work to MLB
RT: Block DT, first step left foot
TE: Block DE, then release to crossing route behind linebackers
TH: Stalk block CB, then release to 5-yard corner route
QB: Receive snap, reverse pivot, make eye contact with HB, lead HB by two steps with pitch
FB: First step left, lead HB around end, picking up first unblocked defender, likely DE
HB: First step left, get horizontal separation from QB, watch pitch into hands, tuck ball as if running 29, then throw to open receiver

PITCH SERIES

Strong Right 28 Pitch Reverse

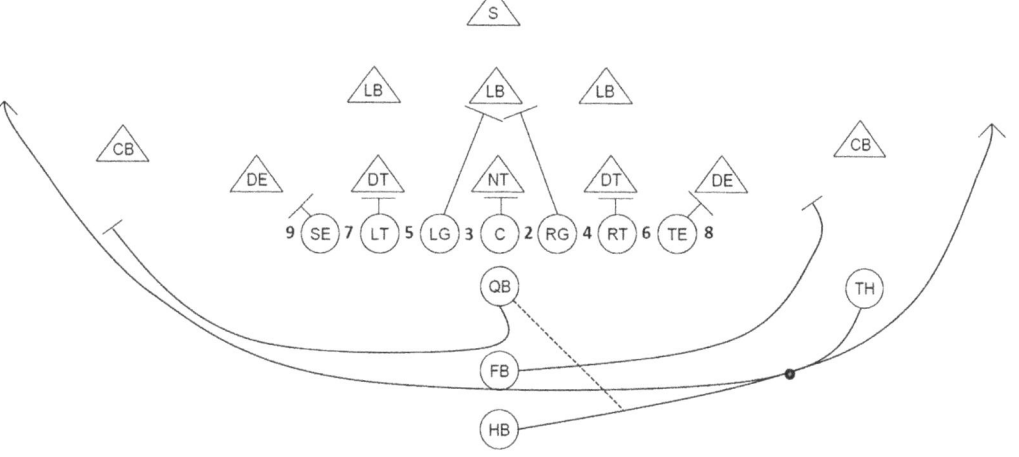

- **SE:** Block DE, first step left foot
- **LT:** Block DT, first step left foot
- **LG:** Chip NT with right arm, work to MLB
- **C:** Block NT
- **RG:** Chip NT with left arm, work to MLB
- **RT:** Block DT, first step left foot
- **TE:** Block DE, first step left foot
- **TH:** First step left foot, orbit path running opposite direction of FB and HB, receive handoff from HB, follow lead block of QB around left end
- **QB:** Receive snap, reverse pivot, make eye contact with HB, lead HB by two steps with pitch, then lead TH around left end
- **FB:** First step right, lead HB around end, picking up first unblocked defender, likely OLB or CB
- **HB:** First step left, get horizontal separation from QB, watch pitch into hands, after securing ball hand off to TH with inside hand, carry out fake around right end

PITCH SERIES

Slots 38 Pitch

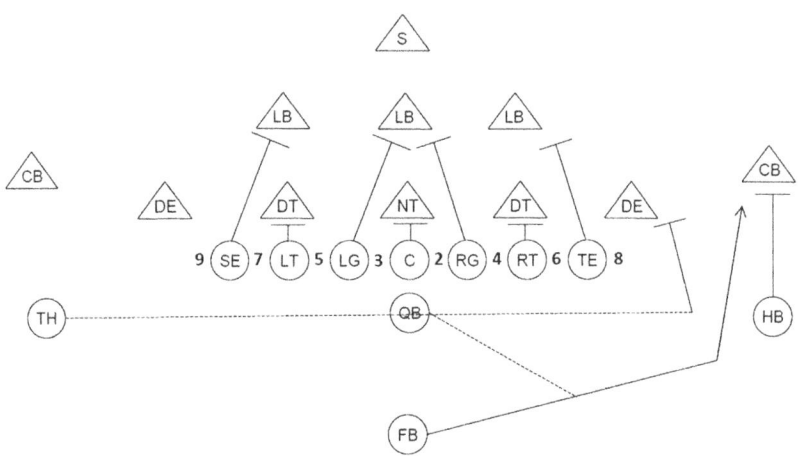

SE: Block OLB, first step left foot
LT: Block DT, first step right foot
LG: Chip NT with right arm, work to MLB
C: Block NT
RG: Chip NT with left arm, work to MLB
RT: Block DT, first step right foot
TE: Block OLB, first step right foot
TH: Go in motion parallel to line of scrimmage, behind QB, on "ready," lead FB around right end after snap, block DE
QB: Receive snap, reverse pivot, make eye contact with FB, lead FB by two steps with pitch
FB: First step right, get horizontal separation from QB, watch pitch into hands, follow TH lead around right end
HB: Stalk block CB or double team DE with TH

PITCH SERIES

Slots 38 Bootleg Pass

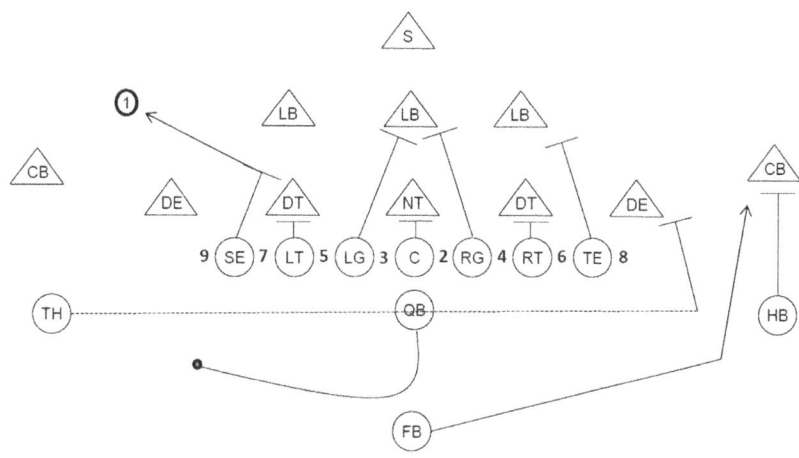

SE: First step right foot, faking block on OLB, then cut off right foot to corner route behind CB

LT: Block DT, first step right foot

LG: Chip NT with right arm, work to MLB

C: Block NT

RG: Chip NT with left arm, work to MLB

RT: Block DT, first step right foot

TE: Block OLB, first step right foot

TH: Go in motion parallel to line of scrimmage, behind QB, on "ready," lead FB around right end after snap, block DE

QB: Receive snap, reverse pivot, make eye contact with FB, fake pitch to FB, make tight turn (no deeper than 3 yards), take 2-3 additional steps, set feet, throw to open receiver

FB: First step right, get horizontal separation from QB, fake pitch into hands, follow TH lead around end

HB: Stalk block CB or double team DE with TH

PITCH SERIES

Slots 39 Pitch

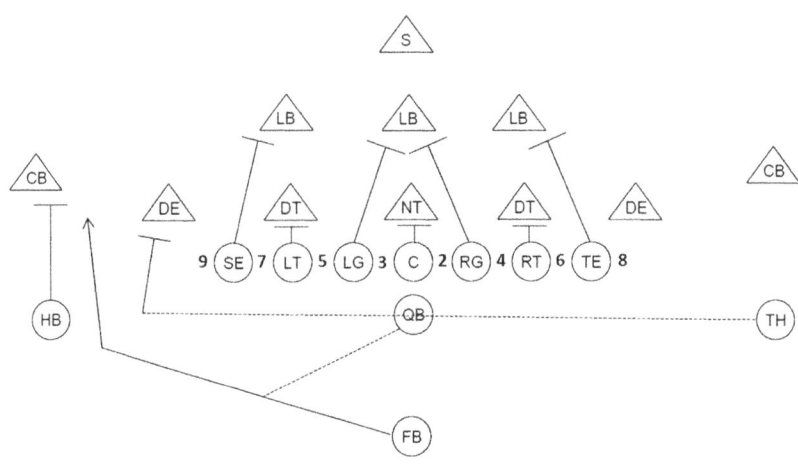

SE: Block OLB, first step left foot
LT: Block DT, first step left foot
LG: Chip NT with right arm, work to MLB
C: Block NT
RG: Chip NT with left arm, work to MLB
RT: Block DT, first step left foot
TE: Block OLB, first step left foot
TH: Go in motion parallel to line of scrimmage, behind QB, on "ready," lead FB around left end after snap, block DE
QB: Receive snap, reverse pivot, make eye contact with FB, lead FB by two steps with pitch
FB: First step left, get horizontal separation from QB, watch pitch into hands, follow TH lead around left end
HB: Stalk block CB or double team DE with TH

PITCH SERIES

Slots 39 Bootleg Pass

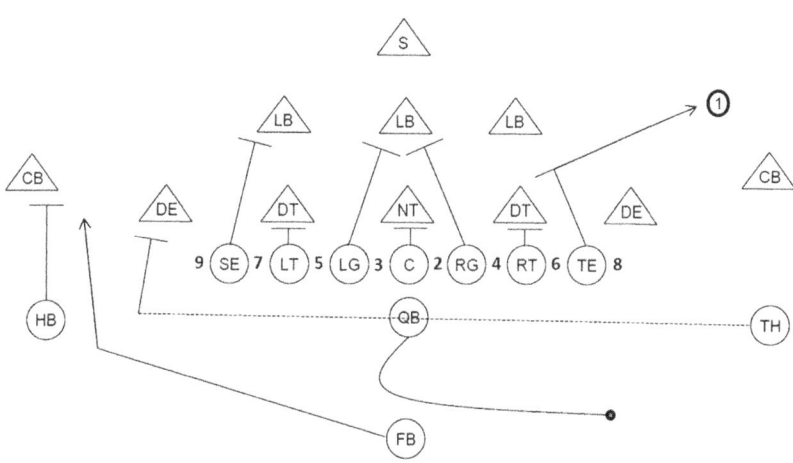

SE: Block OLB, first step left foot
LT: Block DT, first step left foot
LG: Chip NT with right arm, work to MLB
C: Block NT
RG: Chip NT with left arm, work to MLB
RT: Block DT, first step left foot
TE: First step left foot, faking block on OLB, then cut off left foot to corner route behind CB
TH: Go in motion parallel to line of scrimmage, behind QB, on "ready," lead FB around right end after snap, block DE
QB: Receive snap, reverse pivot, make eye contact with FB, fake pitch to FB, make tight turn (no deeper than 3 yards), take 2-3 additional steps, set feet, throw to open receiver
FB: First step right, get horizontal separation from QB, watch pitch into hands, follow TH lead around left end
HB: Stalk block CB or double team DE with TH

PITCH SERIES

Slots 28 Pitch

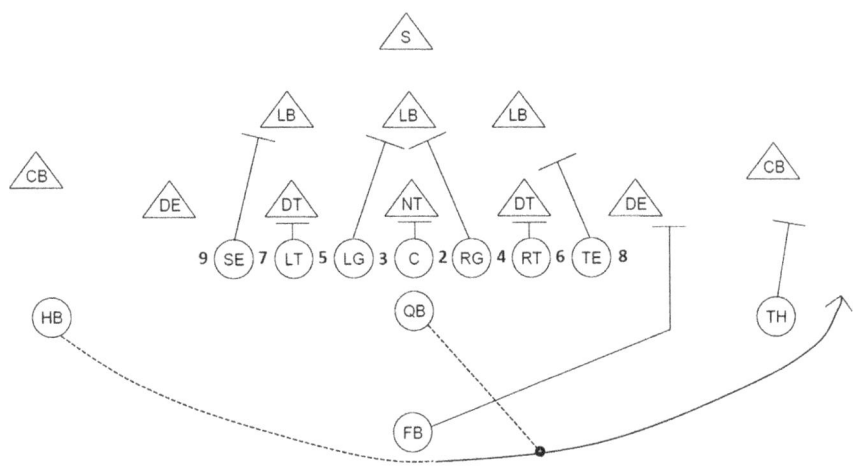

SE: Block OLB, first step left foot
LT: Block DT, first step right foot
LG: Chip NT with right arm, work to MLB
C: Block NT
RG: Chip NT with left arm, work to MLB
RT: Block DT, first step right foot
TE: Block OLB, first step right foot
TH: Stalk block CB or double team DE
QB: Receive snap, reverse pivot, make eye contact with HB, lead HB by two steps with pitch
FB: First step right foot, lead HB around right end, block DE outside shoulder
HB: Go in orbit motion behind FB on "ready," get horizontal separation from QB, watch pitch into hands, follow FB lead around right end

PITCH SERIES

Slots 49 Pitch

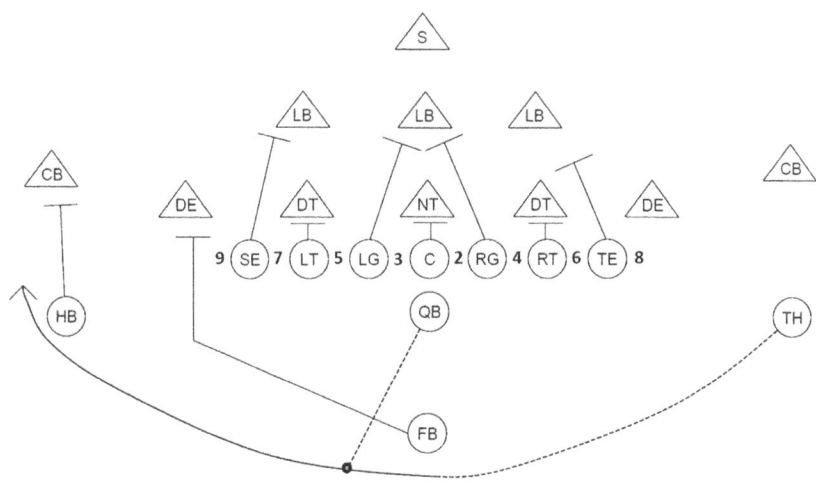

SE: Block OLB, first step left foot
LT: Block DT, first step left foot
LG: Chip NT with right arm, work to MLB
C: Block NT
RG: Chip NT with left arm, work to MLB
RT: Block DT, first step left foot
TE: Block OLB, first step right foot
TH: Go in orbit motion behind FB on "ready," get horizontal separation from QB, watch pitch into hands, follow FB lead around left end
QB: Receive snap, reverse pivot, make eye contact with TH, lead TH by two steps with pitch
FB: First step left foot, lead TH around left end, block DE outside shoulder
HB: Stalk block CB or double team DE

PITCH SERIES

Steamroller Right 48 Pitch

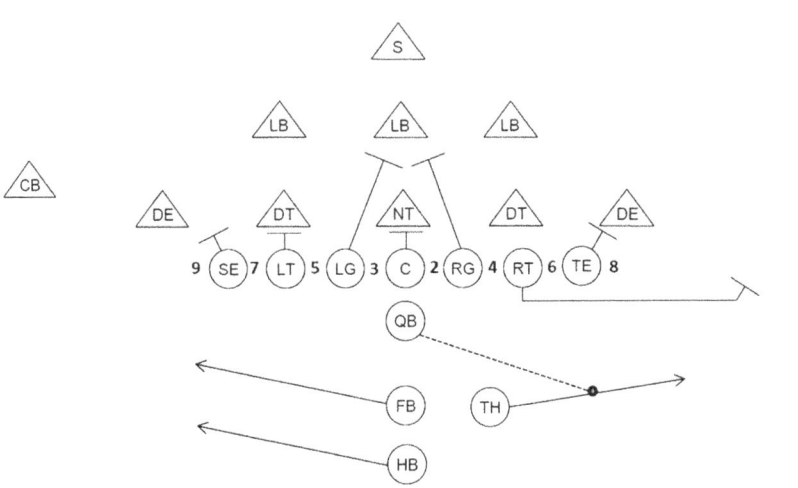

SE: Block DE, first step right foot
LT: Block DT, first step right foot
LG: Chip NT with right arm, work to MLB
C: Block NT
RG: Chip NT with left arm, work to MLB
RT: Bucket step with right foot, turn shoulders toward sideline and pull, square up and lead around right end, pick up first unblocked defender, likely OLB or CB
TE: Block DE, first step right foot
TH: First step right foot, get horizontal separation from QB, watch pitch into hands, follow RT lead around right end
QB: Receive snap, reverse pivot, make eye contact with TH, lead TH by two steps with pitch
FB: First step left foot, fake lead block around left end
HB: First step left foot, fake pitch around left end

PITCH SERIES

Steamroller Left 39 Pitch

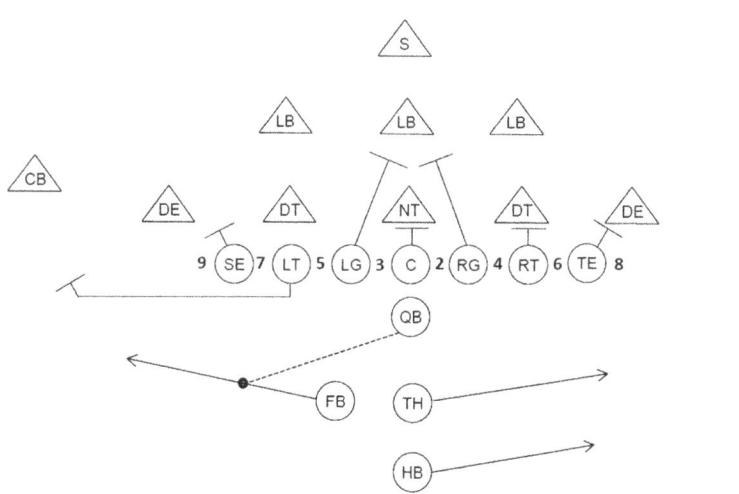

SE: Block DE, first step left foot
LT: Bucket step with left foot, turn shoulders toward sideline and pull, square up and lead around left end, pick up first unblocked defender, likely OLB or CB
LG: Chip NT with right arm, work to MLB
C: Block NT
RG: Chip NT with left arm, work to MLB
RT: Block DT, first step left foot
TE: Block DE, first step left foot
TH: First step right foot, fake lead block around right end
QB: Receive snap, reverse pivot, make eye contact with FB, lead FB by two steps with pitch
FB: First step left foot, get horizontal separation from QB, watch pitch into hands, follow LT lead around left end
HB: First step right foot, fake pitch around right end

QUICK SERIES

Strong Right 11 Sneak

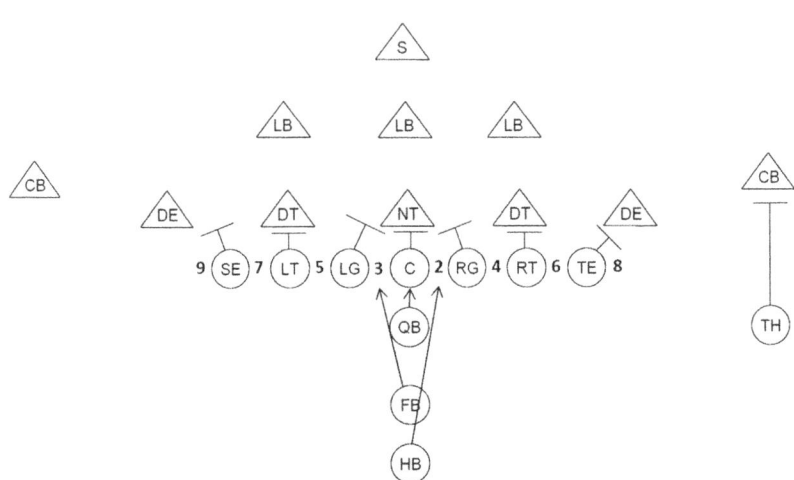

SE: Block DE, first step right foot
LT: Block DT, first step right foot
LG: Triple team NT with C
C: Block NT
RG: Triple team NT with C
RT: Block DT, first step left foot
TE: Block DE, first step left foot
TH: Stalk block CB
QB: After receiving snap follow C straight ahead
FB: First step left foot, watch for fumble
HB: First step right foot, watch for fumble

QUICK SERIES

Strong Right 12 Sneak

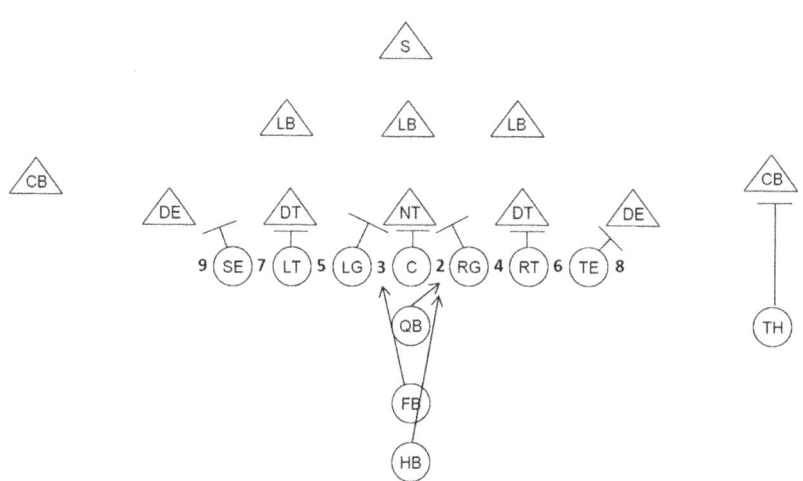

SE: Block DE, first step right foot
LT: Block DT, first step right foot
LG: Triple team NT with C
C: Block NT
RG: Triple team NT with C
RT: Block DT, first step left foot
TE: Block DE, first step left foot
TH: Stalk block CB
QB: After receiving snap run through 2 hole off C right hip
FB: First step left foot, watch for fumble
HB: First step right foot, watch for fumble

QUICK SERIES

Strong Right 33 Dive

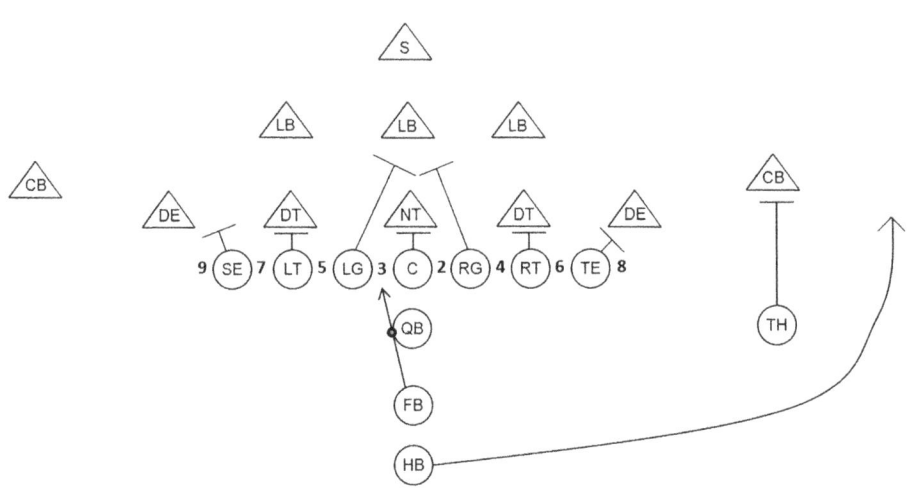

SE: Block DE, first step right foot
LT: Block DT, first step right foot
LG: Chip NT with right arm before climbing to MLB
C: Block NT
RG: Chip NT with left arm before climbing to MLB
RT: Block DT, first step left foot
TE: Block DT, first step left foot
TH: Stalk block CB or double team DE with TE
QB: Quick pivot left, stick ball in FB belly, reverse pivot, fake pitch to HB
FB: First step left foot, arms ready to receive handoff immediately, run through 3 hole
HB: First step right foot, fake pitch around right end

QUICK SERIES

Strong Right 33 Fake 28 Pitch

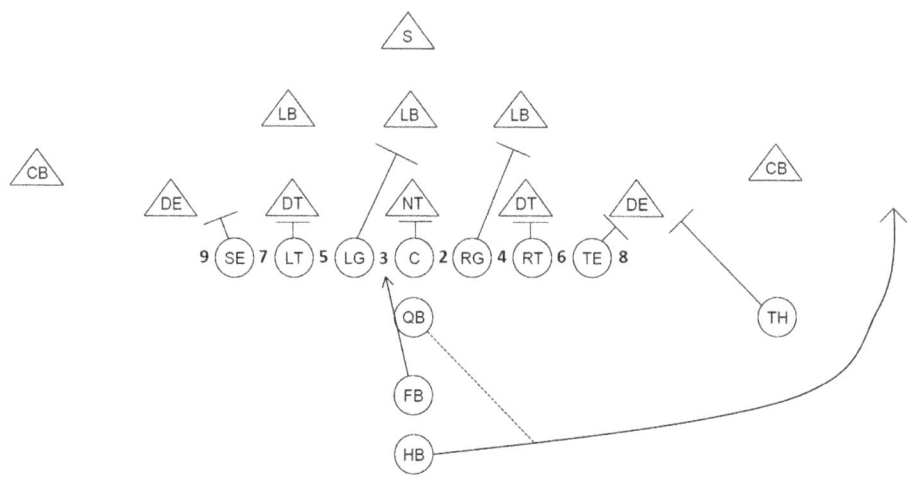

SE: Block DE, first step right foot
LT: Block DT, first step right foot
LG: Chip NT with right arm before climbing to MLB
C: Block NT
RG: Chip NT with left arm before climbing to OLB
RT: Block DT, first step left foot
TE: Block DT, first step left foot
TH: Double team DE with TE or stalk block CB
QB: Quick pivot left, stick ball in FB belly, remove, reverse pivot, pitch to HB, leading by two steps with pitch
FB: First step left foot, arms ready to receive handoff immediately, carry out fake through 3 hole
HB: First step right, get horizontal separation from QB, watch pitch into hands, run around right end

QUICK SERIES

Strong Left 33 Fake Option Left

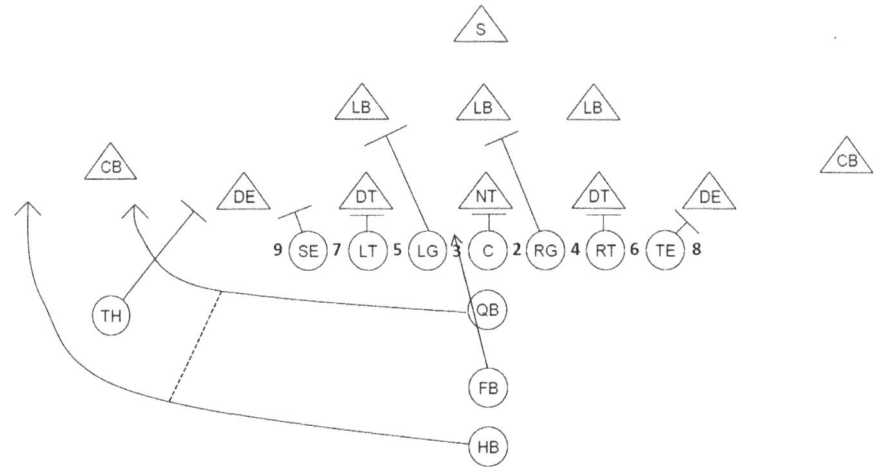

SE: Block DE, first step left foot
LT: Block DT, first step left foot
LG: Chip NT with right arm before climbing to OLB
C: Block NT
RG: Chip NT with left arm before climbing to MLB
RT: Block DT, first step left foot
TE: Block DT, first step left foot
TH: Double team DE with TE
QB: Quick pivot left, stick ball in FB belly, remove, run parallel to line of scrimmage, read CB to keep and cut back or pitch to HB
FB: First step left foot, arms ready to receive handoff immediately, carry out fake through 3 hole
HB: First step left, get horizontal separation from QB, maintain 3-5 yard pitch relationship with QB as he runs parallel to line of scrimmage, hands ready to receive pitch based on CB read

QUICK SERIES

Strong Right 33 Fake SE Pass

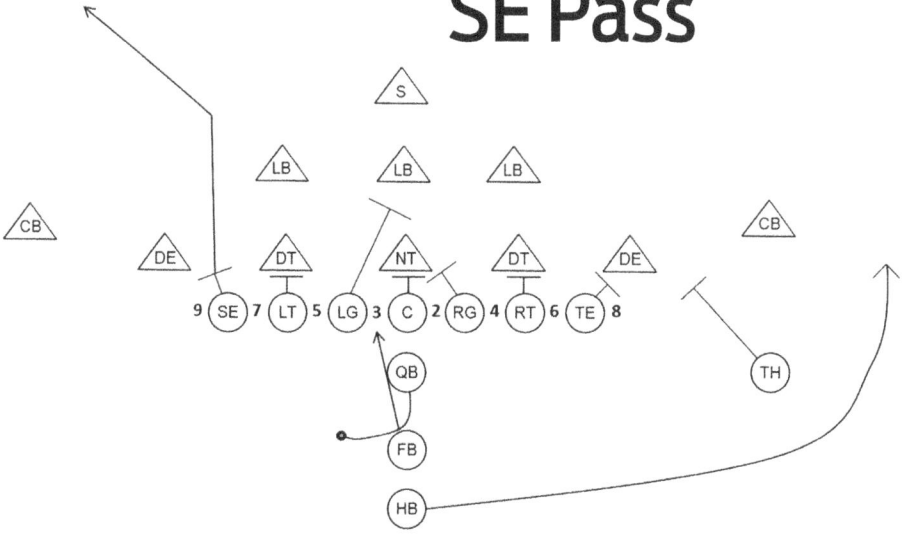

SE: Block DE, first step right foot, then release to 5-yard corner route, cutting off right foot

LT: Block DT, first step right foot

LG: Chip NT with right arm before climbing to MLB

C: Block NT

RG: Double team NT with C

RT: Block DT, first step left foot

TE: Block DE, first step left foot

TH: Double team DE with TE

QB: Quick pivot left, stick ball in FB belly, remove, take 2-3 additional steps, set feet, throw to open receiver

FB: First step left foot, arms ready to receive handoff immediately, carry out fake through 3 hole

HB: First step right foot, fake pitch around right end

QUICK SERIES

Strong Left 32 Dive

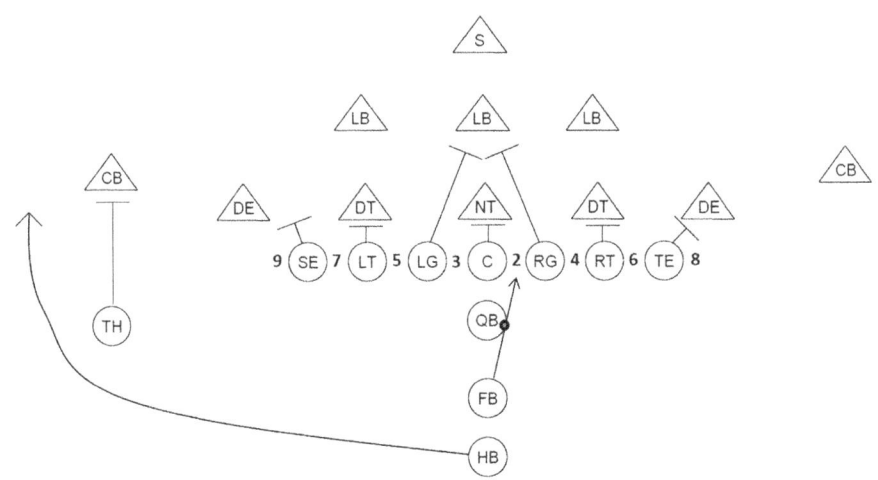

SE: Block DE, first step right foot
LT: Block DT, first step right foot
LG: Chip NT with right arm before climbing to MLB
C: Block NT
RG: Chip NT with left arm before climbing to MLB
RT: Block DT, first step left foot
TE: Block DT, first step left foot
TH: Stalk block CB or double team DE with SE
QB: Quick pivot right, stick ball in FB belly, reverse pivot, fake pitch to HB
FB: First step right foot, arms ready to receive handoff immediately, run through 2 hole
HB: First step left foot, fake pitch around left end

QUICK SERIES

Strong Left 32 Fake 29 Pitch

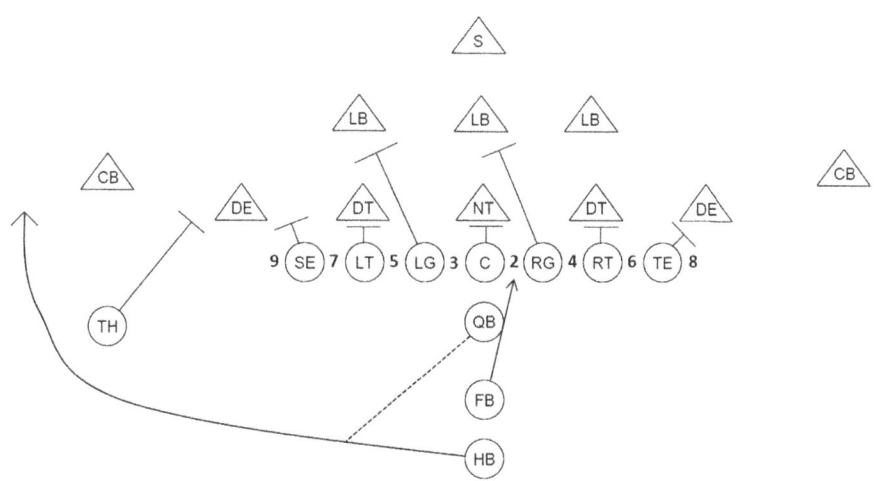

SE: Block DE, first step right foot
LT: Block DT, first step right foot
LG: Chip NT with right arm before climbing to MLB
C: Block NT
RG: Chip NT with left arm before climbing to OLB
RT: Block DT, first step left foot
TE: Block DT, first step left foot
TH: Double team DE with SE or stalk block CB
QB: Quick pivot right, stick ball in FB belly, remove, reverse pivot, pitch to HB, leading by two steps with pitch
FB: First step right foot, arms ready to receive handoff immediately, carry out fake through 2 hole
HB: First step left, get horizontal separation from QB, watch pitch into hands, run around left end

QUICK SERIES

Strong Right 32 Fake Option Right

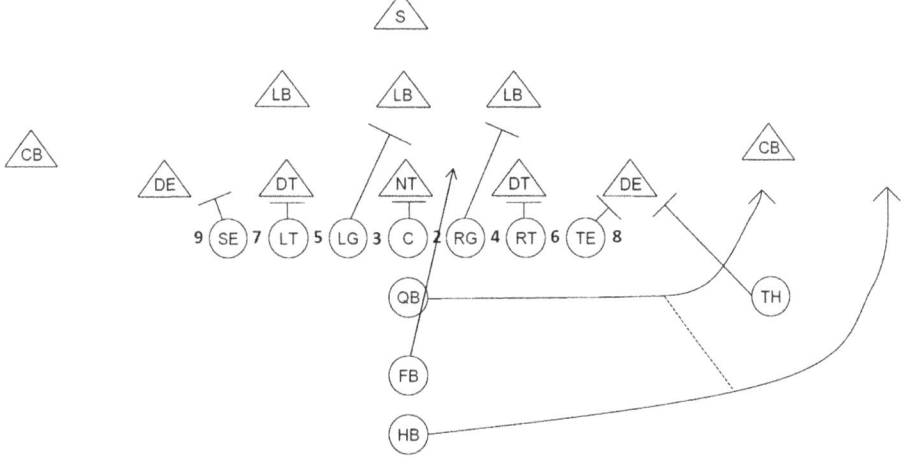

SE: Block DE, first step right foot

LT: Block DT, first step right foot

LG: Chip NT with right arm before climbing to MLB

C: Block NT

RG: Chip NT with left arm before climbing to OLB

RT: Block DT, first step right foot

TE: Block DT, first step right foot

TH: Double team DE with TE

QB: Quick pivot right, stick ball in FB belly, remove, run parallel to line of scrimmage, read CB to keep and cut back or pitch to HB

FB: First step right foot, arms ready to receive handoff immediately, carry out fake through 2 hole

HB: First step right, get horizontal separation from QB, maintain 3-5 yard pitch relationship with QB as he runs parallel to line of scrimmage, hands ready to receive pitch based on CB read

QUICK SERIES

Strong Left 32 Fake TE Pass

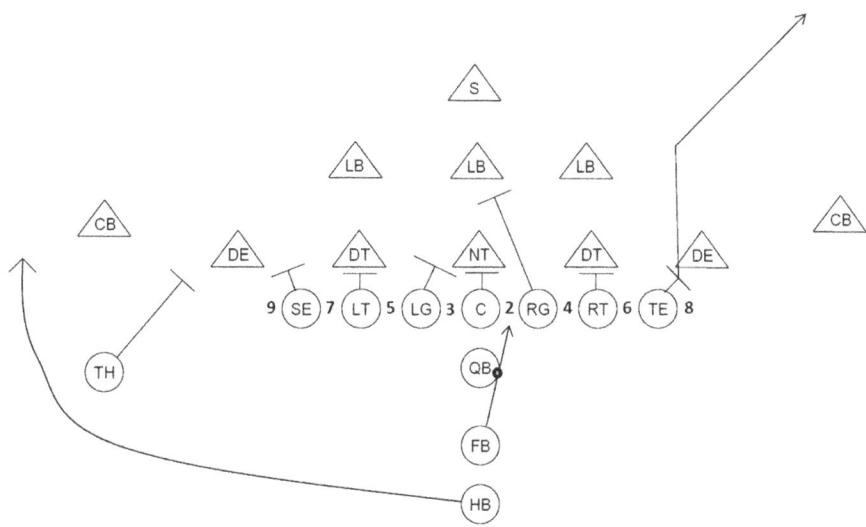

SE: Block DE, first step right foot

LT: Block DT, first step right foot

LG: Double team NT with C

C: Block NT

RG: Chip NT with left arm before climbing to MLB

RT: Block DT, first step left foot

TE: Block DE, first step left foot, then release to 5-yard corner route, cutting off left foot

TH: Double team DE with SE

QB: Quick pivot right, stick ball in FB belly, remove, take 2-3 additional steps, set feet, throw to open receiver

FB: First step right foot, arms ready to receive handoff immediately, carry out fake through 2 hole

HB: First step left foot, fake pitch around left end

QUICK SERIES

Pro Right 35 Dive

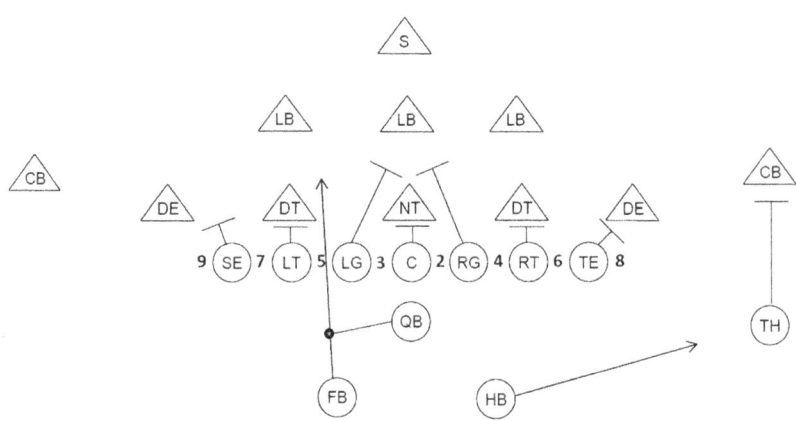

- **SE:** Block DE, first step right foot
- **LT:** Block DT, first step right foot
- **LG:** Chip NT with right arm before climbing to MLB
- **C:** Block NT
- **RG:** Chip NT with left arm before climbing to MLB
- **RT:** Block DT, first step left foot
- **TE:** Block DE, first step left foot
- **TH:** Stalk block CB
- **QB:** Pivot left, meet FB behind 5 hole for handoff
- **FB:** First step left foot, arms ready to receive handoff immediately, run through 5 hole
- **HB:** First step right foot, fake pitch around right end

QUICK SERIES

Pro Right 24 Dive

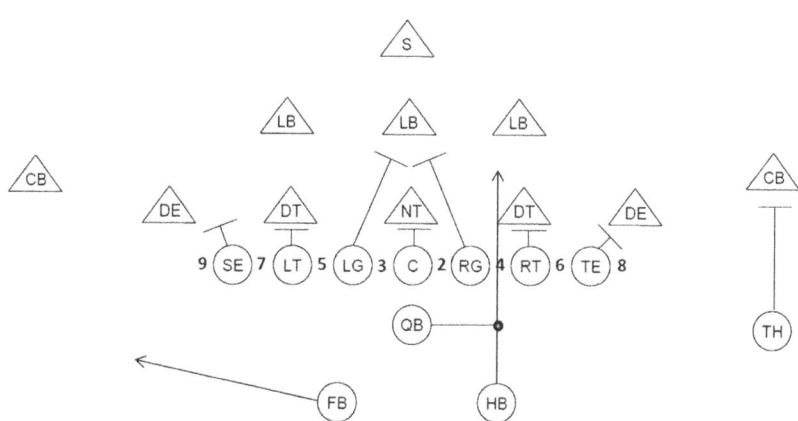

SE: Block DE, first step right foot
LT: Block DT, first step right foot
LG: Chip NT with right arm before climbing to MLB
C: Block NT
RG: Chip NT with left arm before climbing to MLB
RT: Block DT, first step left foot
TE: Block DE, first step left foot
TH: Stalk block CB
QB: Pivot right, meet HB behind 4 hole for handoff
FB: First step left foot, fake pitch around left end
HB: First step right foot, arms ready to receive handoff immediately, run through 4 hole

QUICK SERIES

T 35 Dive

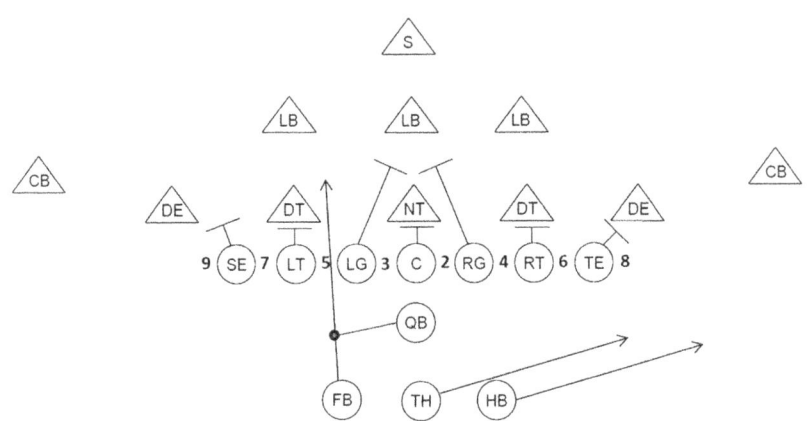

SE: Block DE, first step right foot
LT: Block DT, first step right foot
LG: Chip NT with right arm before climbing to MLB
C: Block NT
RG: Chip NT with left arm before climbing to MLB
RT: Block DT, first step left foot
TE: Block DE, first step left foot
TH: Fake lead block around right end
QB: Pivot left, meet FB behind 5 hole for handoff
FB: First step left foot, arms ready to receive handoff immediately, run through 5 hole
HB: First step right foot, fake pitch around right end

QUICK SERIES

T 42 Dive

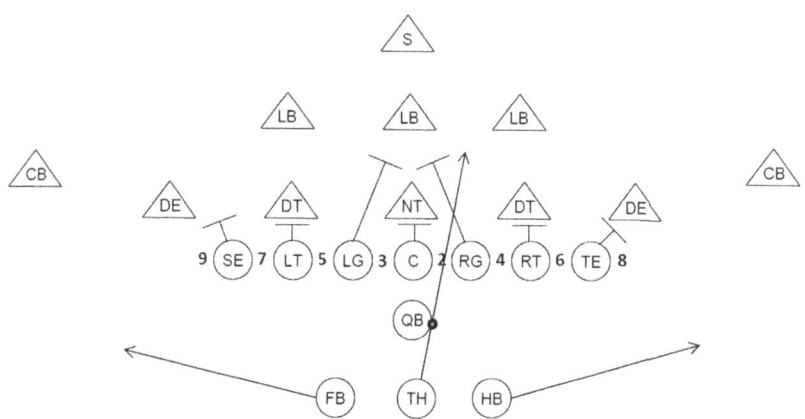

SE: Block DE, first step right foot
LT: Block DT, first step right foot
LG: Chip NT with right arm before climbing to MLB
C: Block NT
RG: Chip NT with left arm before climbing to MLB
RT: Block DT, first step left foot
TE: Block DE, first step left foot
TH: First step right foot, arms ready to receive handoff immediately, run through 2 hole
QB: Pivot right, quick handoff to TH behind 2 hole
FB: First step left foot, fake pitch around left end
HB: First step right foot, fake pitch around right end

QUICK SERIES

T 24 Dive

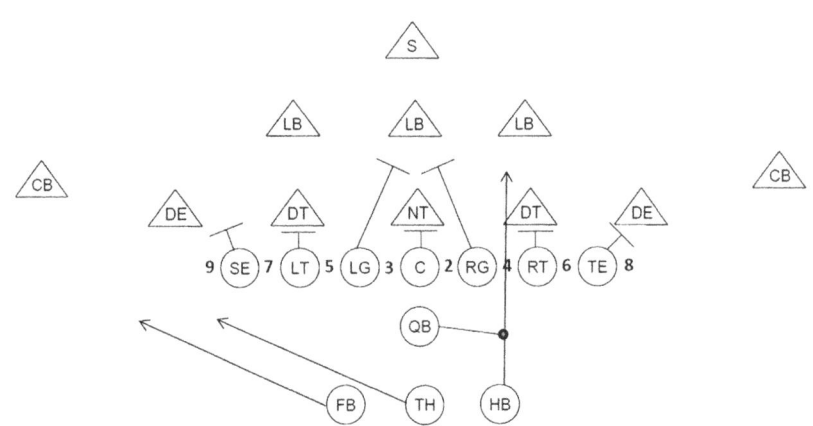

SE: Block DE, first step right foot
LT: Block DT, first step right foot
LG: Chip NT with right arm before climbing to MLB
C: Block NT
RG: Chip NT with left arm before climbing to MLB
RT: Block DT, first step left foot
TE: Block DE, first step left foot
TH: Fake lead block around left end
QB: Pivot right, meet HB behind 4 hole for handoff
FB: First step left foot, fake pitch around left end
HB: First step right foot, arms ready to receive handoff immediately, run through 4 hole

QUICK SERIES

Strong Right Pop Pass

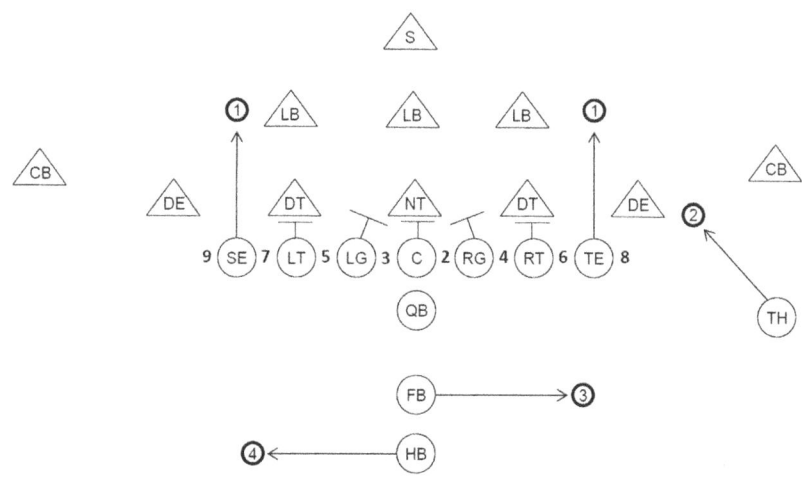

SE: First step left foot, immediately snap head over right shoulder and look for pass
LT: Pass block
LG: Pass block
C: Pass block
RG: Pass block
RT: Pass block
TE: First step right foot, immediately snap head over left shoulder and look for pass
TH: First step left foot, run quick slant in front of CB
QB: Receive snap, three-step drop, pass to open receiver
FB: First step right foot, flare to right
HB: First step left foot, flare to left

QUICK SERIES

Slots Quick Hit

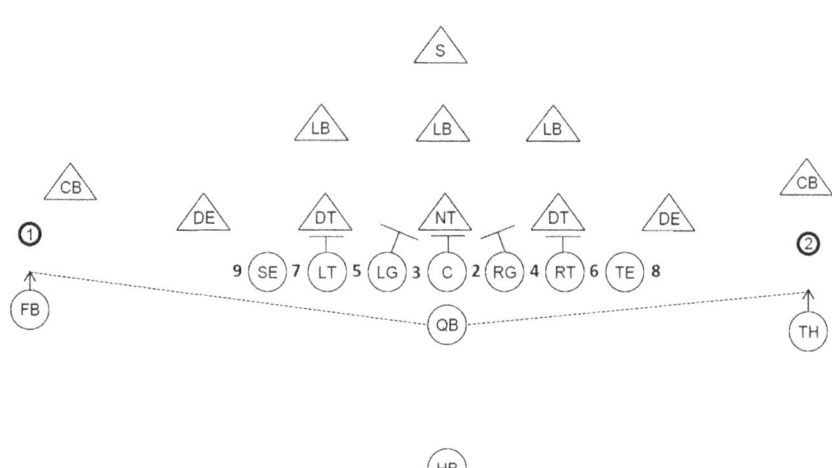

SE: Pass block
LT: Pass block
LG: Pass block
C: Pass block
RG: Pass block
RT: Pass block
TE: Pass block
TH: At snap turn and face QB, hands ready for pass
QB: Receive snap, turn shoulders toward predetermined receiver, make throw
FB: At snap turn and face QB, hands ready for pass
HB: Pass block

QUICK SERIES

Slots Two Verticals

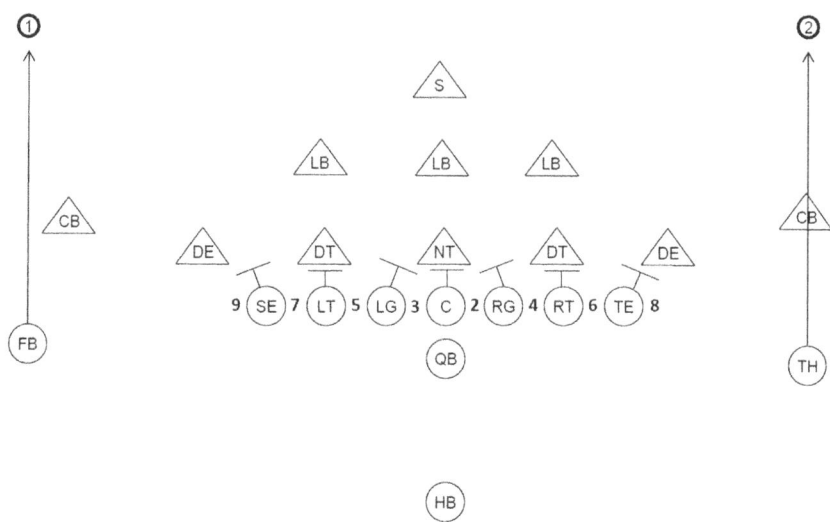

SE: Pass block
LT: Pass block
LG: Pass block
C: Pass block
RG: Pass block
RT: Pass block
TE: Pass block
TH: Run go route, snapping head over left shoulder after 10 yards to look for pass
QB: Receive snap, five-step drop, turn shoulders toward predetermined receiver, make throw
FB: Run go route, snapping head over right shoulder after 10 yards to look for pass
HB: Pass block

QUICK SERIES

Slots Two Slants

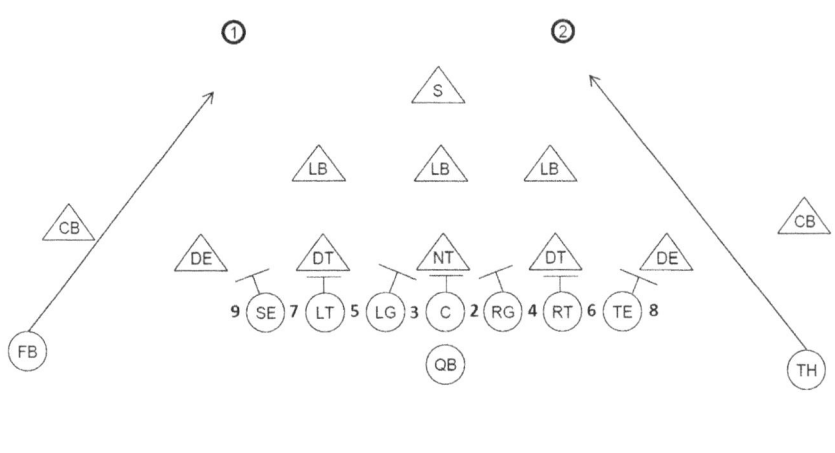

SE: Pass block
LT: Pass block
LG: Pass block
C: Pass block
RG: Pass block
RT: Pass block
TE: Pass block
TH: Run slant in front of CB
QB: Receive snap, five-step drop, turn shoulders toward predetermined receiver, make throw
FB: Run slant in front of CB
HB: Pass block

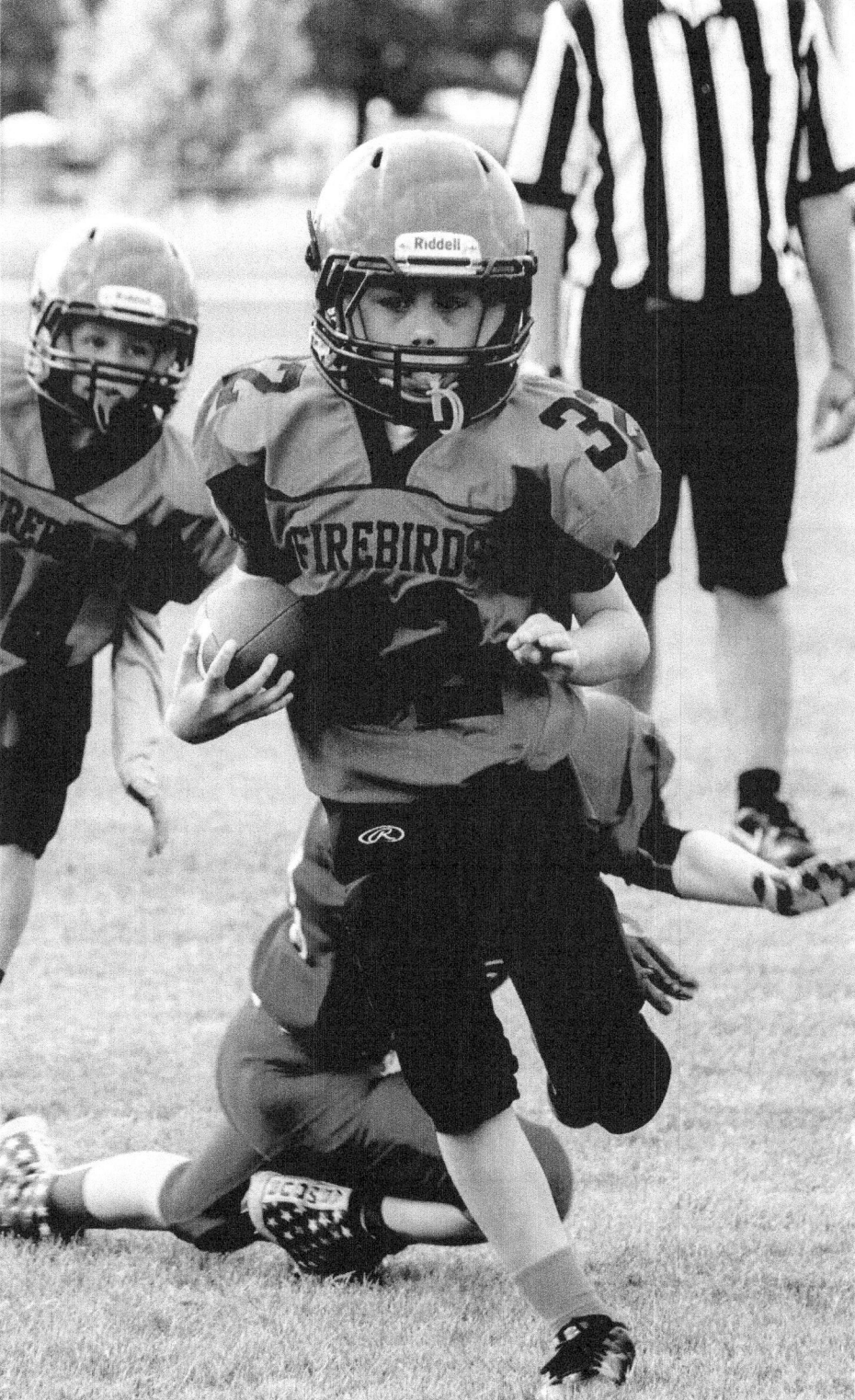

KEEPER SERIES

Strong Right 18 Sweep

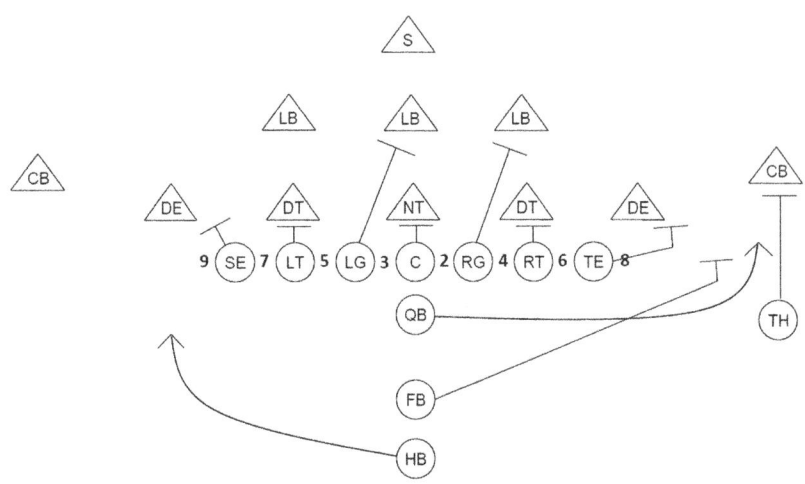

SE: Block DE, first step right foot
LT: Block DT, first step right foot
LG: Chip NT with right arm, climb to MLB
C: Block NT
RG: Chip NT with left arm, climb to OLB
RT: Block DT, first step right foot
TE: Block DE, first step right foot
TH: Stalk block CB or double team DE
QB: Bucket step right foot, turn shoulders to sideline, run parallel to line of scrimmage, following and cutting off FB block
FB: First step right foot, lead QB around right end
HB: Fake pitch around left end

KEEPER SERIES

Heavy Right 18 Sweep

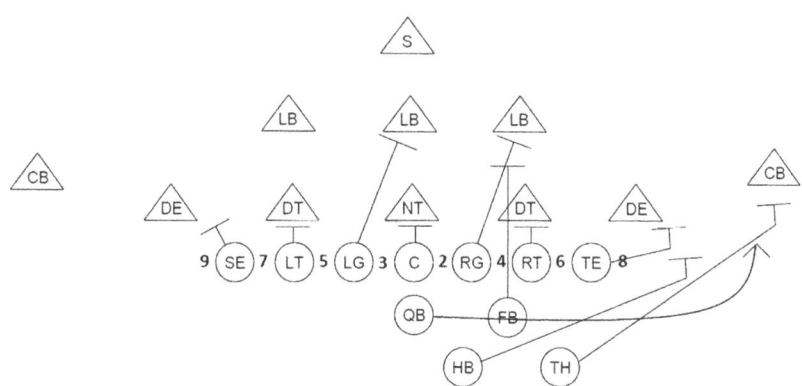

SE: Block DE, first step right foot
LT: Block DT, first step right foot
LG: Chip NT with right arm, climb to MLB
C: Block NT
RG: Chip NT with left arm, climb to OLB
RT: Block DT, first step right foot
TE: Block DE, first step right foot
TH: First step right foot, lead QB to corner, block CB
QB: Bucket step right foot, turn shoulders to sideline, run parallel to line of scrimmage, following and cutting off HB block
FB: First step right foot, run through 4 hole to block OLB or MLB
HB: First step right foot, lead QB around right end

KEEPER SERIES

Strong Right 16 Dive Kick

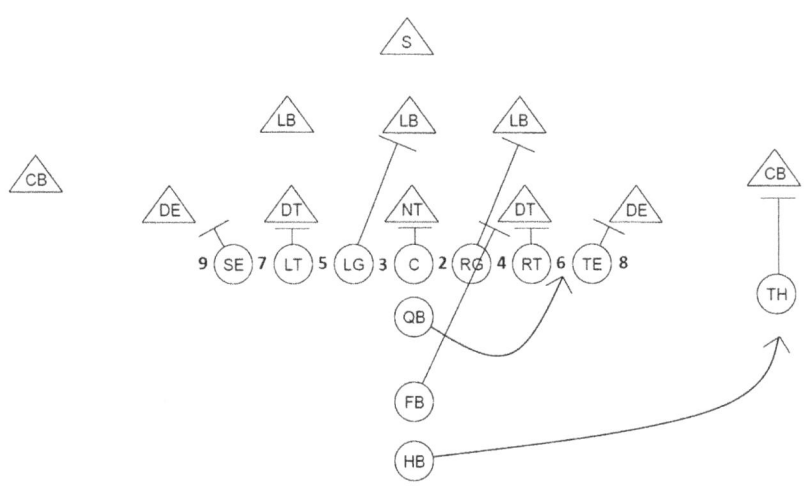

SE: Block DE, first step right foot
LT: Block DT, first step right foot
LG: Chip NT with right arm, climb to MLB
C: Block NT
RG: Chip NT with left arm, climb to OLB
RT: Block DT, first step right foot
TE: Block DE, first step left foot
TH: Stalk block CB or double team DE
QB: Bucket step right foot, turn shoulders to sideline, aim for TE inside hip, run through 6 hole
FB: First step right foot, block DT
HB: First step right foot, fake pitch around right end

KEEPER SERIES

Club Right 110 Sweep

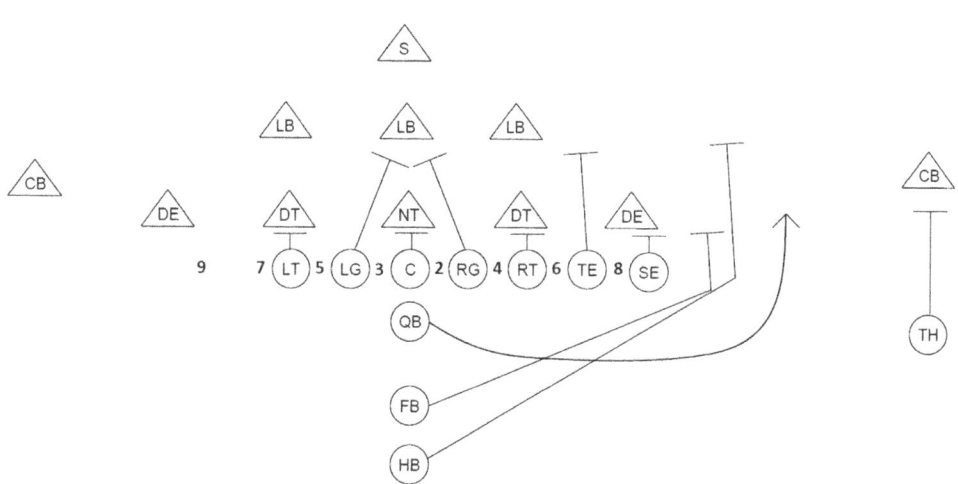

SE: Block DE, first step right foot
LT: Block DT, first step right foot
LG: Chip NT with right arm, climb to MLB
C: Block NT
RG: Chip NT with left arm, climb to MLB
RT: Block DT, first step right foot
TE: Block OLB, first step right foot
TH: Stalk block CB or double team DE
QB: Bucket step right foot, turn shoulders to sideline, run parallel to line of scrimmage, following and cutting off FB, HB blocks
FB: First step right foot, lead QB around right end
HB: First step right foot, lead QB around right end

KEEPER SERIES

Strong Right 18 Reverse

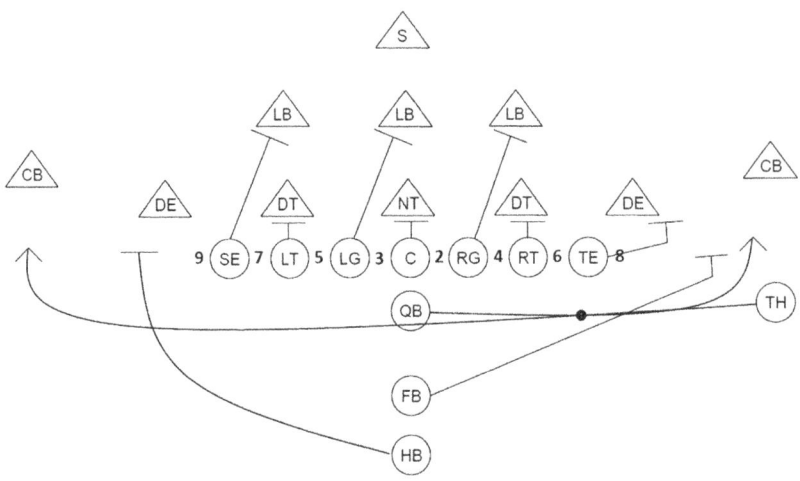

SE: First step left foot, block OLB
LT: Block DT, first step left foot
LG: Chip NT with right arm, climb to MLB
C: Block NT
RG: Chip NT with left arm, climb to OLB
RT: Block DT, first step right foot
TE: Block DE, first step right foot
TH: After snap turn shoulders toward sideline, run parallel to line of scrimmage deeper than QB, take handoff inside, follow HB lead around left end
QB: Bucket step right foot, turn shoulders to sideline, run parallel to line of scrimmage, hand off to TH with outside hand, carry out fake around right end
FB: First step right foot, lead block around right end
HB: First step left foot, lead block around left end, pick up DE

KEEPER SERIES

Strong Right TH Post

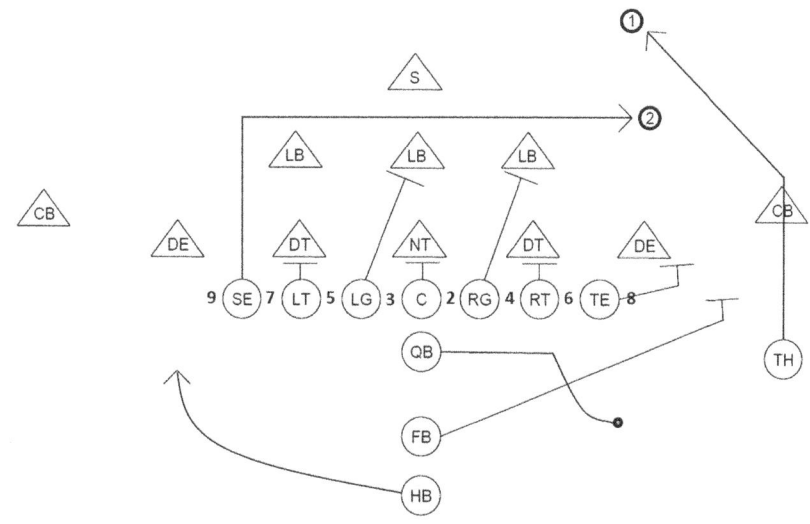

SE: First step left foot, run crossing route behind linebackers
LT: Block DT, first step right foot
LG: Chip NT with right arm, climb to MLB
C: Block NT
RG: Chip NT with left arm, climb to OLB
RT: Block DT, first step right foot
TE: Block DE, first step right foot
TH: Fake stalk block on CB, run 5-yard post route, cutting with right foot
QB: Bucket step right foot, turn shoulders to sideline, run parallel to line of scrimmage, veering back at 4 hole, setting feet and throwing to open receiver
FB: First step right foot, lead block around right end, pick up pass rusher
HB: First step left foot, lead block around left end, pick up pass rusher

KEEPER SERIES

Strong Left 19 Sweep

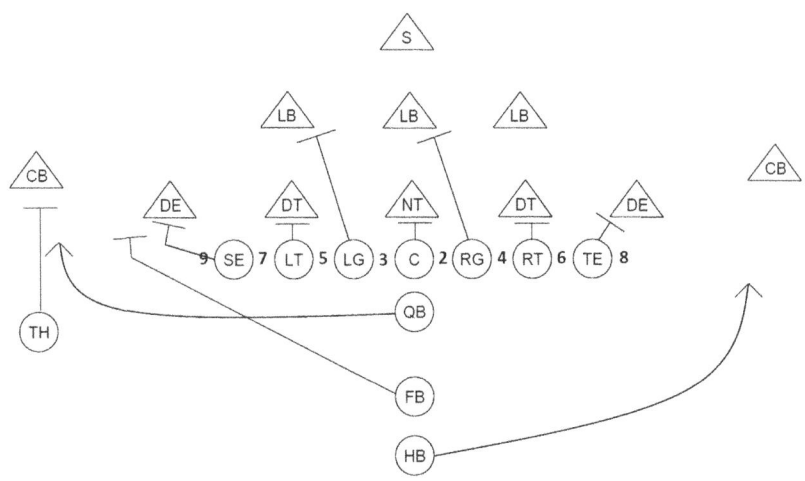

SE: Block DE, first step left foot
LT: Block DT, first step left foot
LG: Chip NT with right arm, climb to OLB
C: Block NT
RG: Chip NT with left arm, climb to MLB
RT: Block DT, first step left foot
TE: Block DE, first step left foot
TH: Stalk block CB or double team DE
QB: Bucket step left foot, turn shoulders to sideline, run parallel to line of scrimmage, following and cutting off FB block
FB: First step left foot, lead QB around left end
HB: Fake pitch around right end

KEEPER SERIES

Heavy Left 19 Sweep

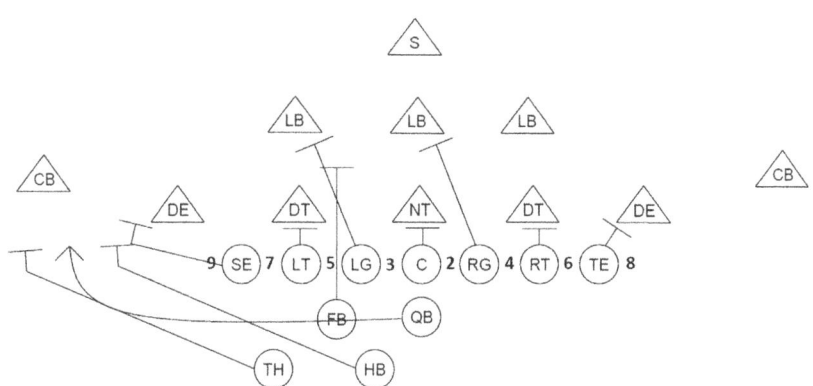

SE: Block DE, first step left foot
LT: Block DT, first step left foot
LG: Chip NT with right arm, climb to OLB
C: Block NT
RG: Chip NT with left arm, climb to MLB
RT: Block DT, first step left foot
TE: Block DE, first step left foot
TH: First step left foot, lead QB to corner, block CB
QB: Bucket step left foot, turn shoulders to sideline, run parallel to line of scrimmage, following and cutting off HB block
FB: First step left foot, run through 5 hole to block OLB or MLB
HB: First step left foot, lead QB around left end

KEEPER SERIES

Strong Left 17 Dive Kick

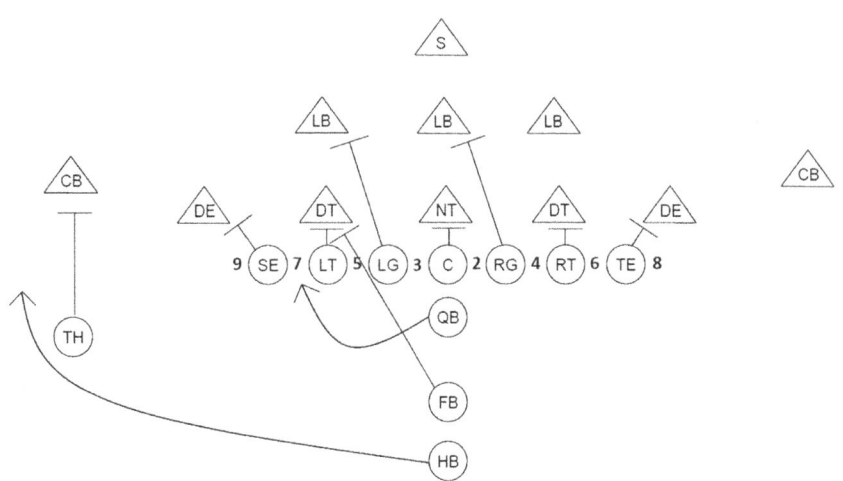

SE: Block DE, first step right foot
LT: Block DT, first step left foot
LG: Chip NT with right arm, climb to OLB
C: Block NT
RG: Chip NT with left arm, climb to MLB
RT: Block DT, first step left foot
TE: Block DE, first step left foot
TH: Stalk block CB or double team DE
QB: Bucket step left foot, turn shoulders to sideline, aim for SE inside hip, run through 7 hole
FB: First step left foot, block DT
HB: First step left foot, fake pitch around left end

KEEPER SERIES

Club Left 111 Sweep

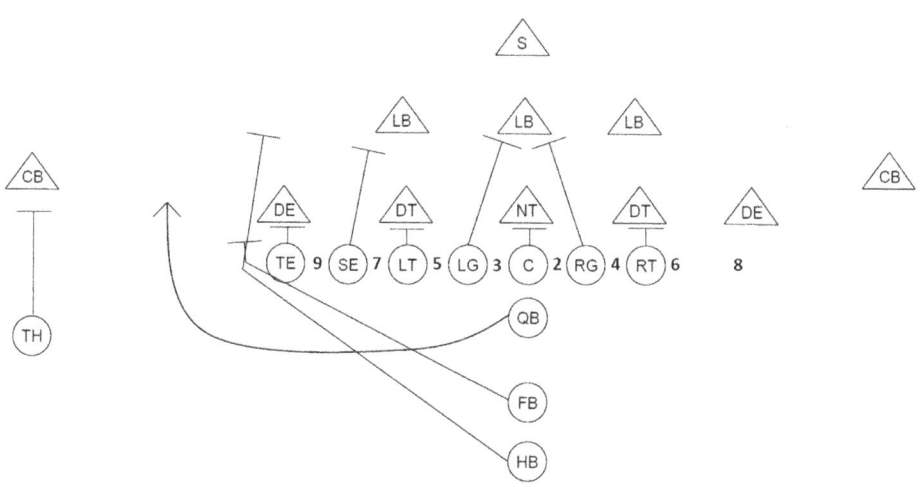

SE: Block OLB, first step left foot
LT: Block DT, first step left foot
LG: Chip NT with right arm, climb to MLB
C: Block NT
RG: Chip NT with left arm, climb to MLB
RT: Block DT, first step left foot
TE: Block DE, first step left foot
TH: Stalk block CB or double team DE
QB: Bucket step left foot, turn shoulders to sideline, run parallel to line of scrimmage, following and cutting off FB, HB blocks
FB: First step left foot, lead QB around left end
HB: First step left foot, lead QB around left end

KEEPER SERIES

Strong Left 19 Reverse

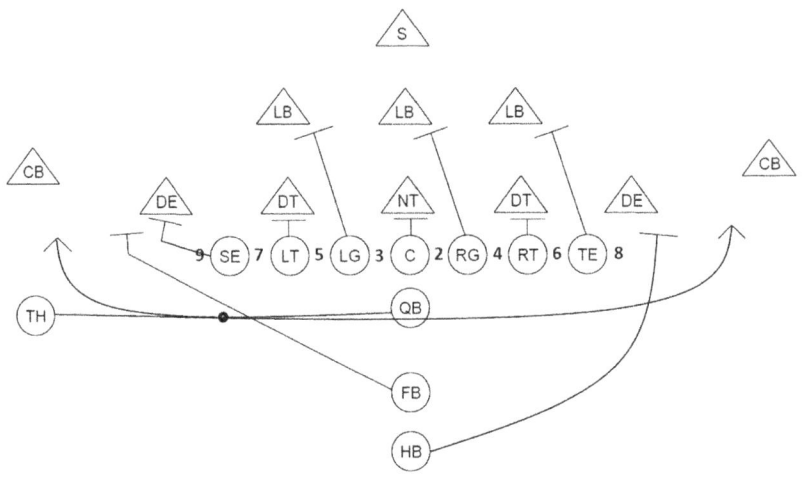

SE: Block DE, first step left foot
LT: Block DT, first step left foot
LG: Chip NT with right arm, climb to OLB
C: Block NT
RG: Chip NT with left arm, climb to MLB
RT: Block DT, first step right foot
TE: First step right foot, block OLB
TH: After snap turn shoulders toward sideline, run parallel to line of scrimmage deeper than QB, take handoff inside, follow HB lead around right end
QB: Bucket step left foot, turn shoulders to sideline, run parallel to line of scrimmage, hand off to TH with outside hand, carry out fake around left end
FB: First step left foot, lead block around left end
HB: First step right foot, lead block around right end, pick up DE

KEEPER SERIES

Strong Left TH Post

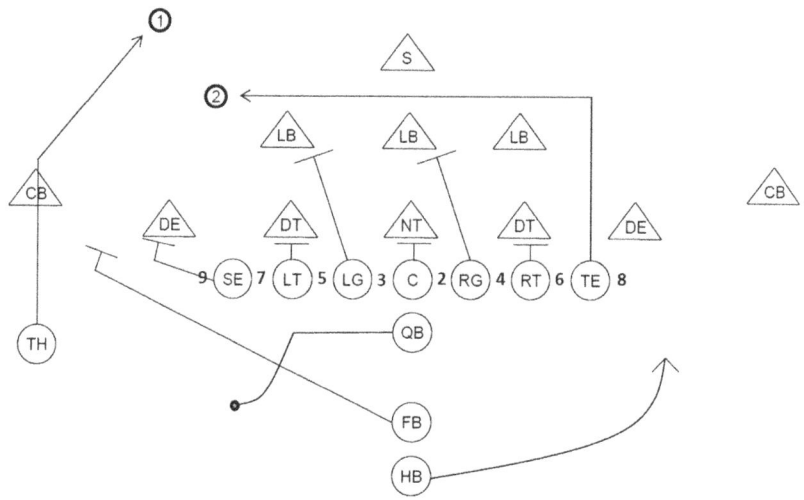

SE: Block DE, first step left foot
LT: Block DT, first step left foot
LG: Chip NT with right arm, climb to OLB
C: Block NT
RG: Chip NT with left arm, climb to MLB
RT: Block DT, first step left foot
TE: First step right foot, run crossing route behind linebackers
TH: Fake stalk block on CB, run 5-yard post route, cutting with left foot
QB: Bucket step left foot, turn shoulders to sideline, run parallel to line of scrimmage, veering back at 5 hole, setting feet and throwing to open receiver
FB: First step left foot, lead block around left end, pick up pass rusher
HB: First step right foot, lead block around right end, pick up pass rusher

KEEPER SERIES

The Barge

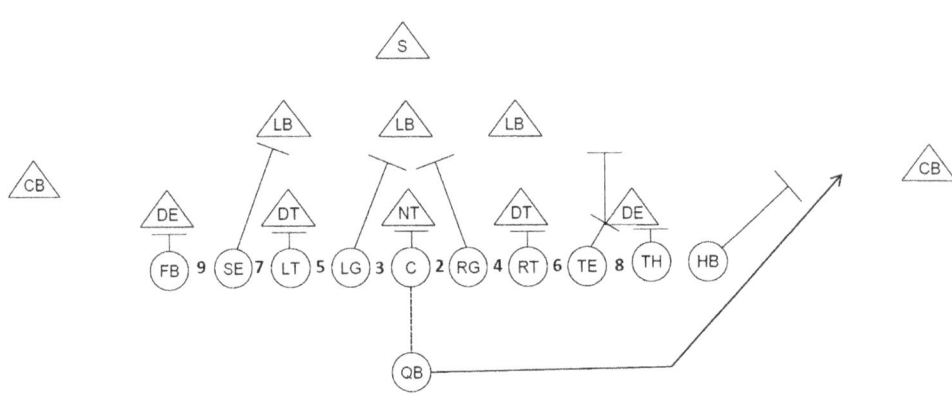

SE: First step left foot, block OLB
LT: Block DT, first step right foot
LG: Chip NT with right arm, climb to MLB
C: Block NT
RG: Chip NT with left arm, climb to MLB
RT: Block DT, first step right foot
TE: Chip DE with right arm, climb to OLB
TH: Block DE, climb to OLB
QB: From shotgun, first step right, choose best hole
FB: Block DE, first step right
HB: Pick up first unblocked defender, first step right

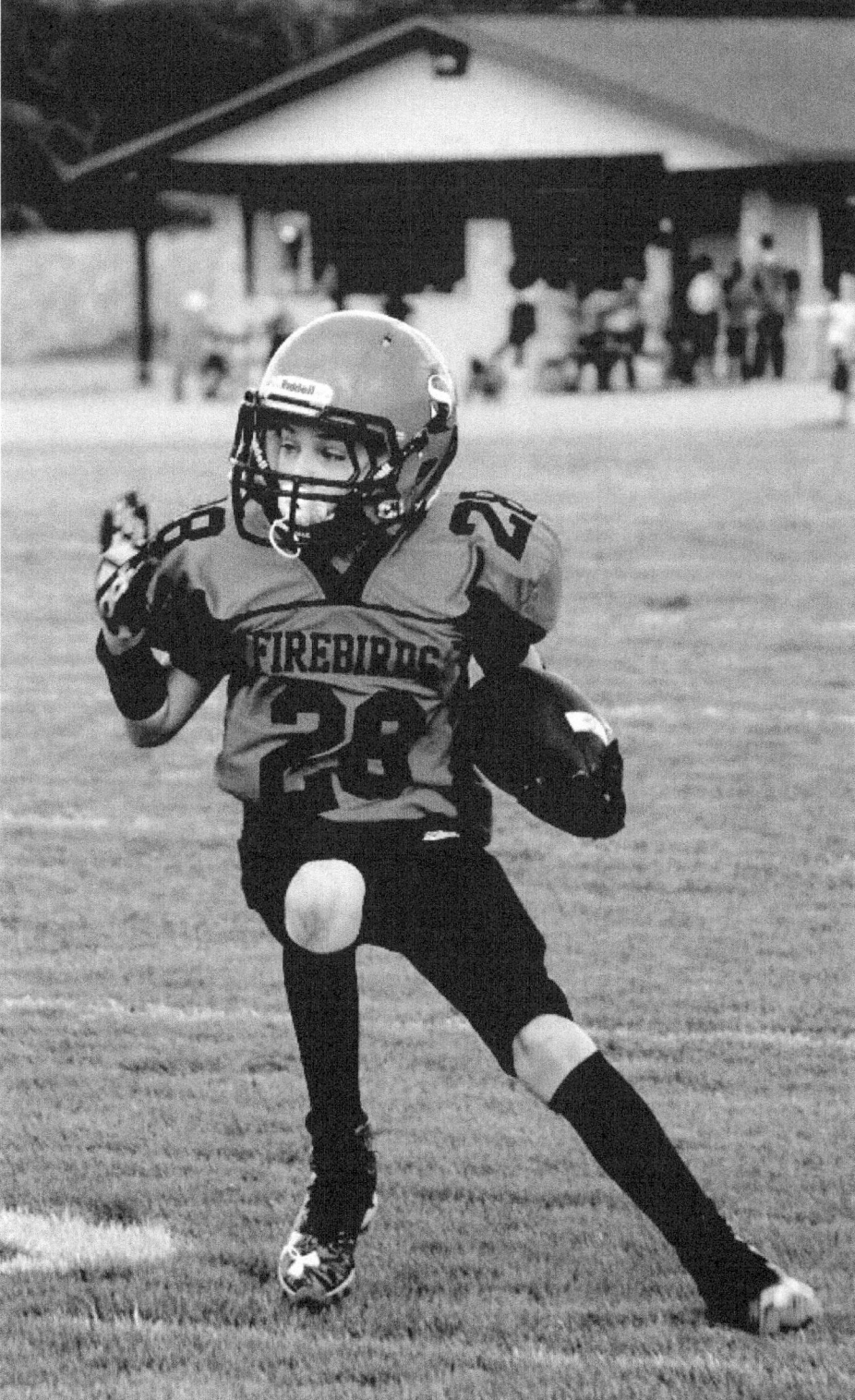

ROCKET SERIES

Slots 48 Jet Sweep

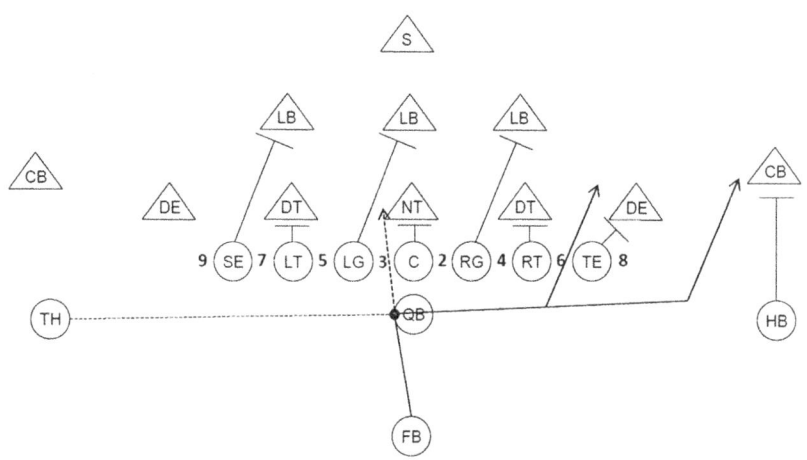

SE: First step left foot, block OLB
LT: Block DT, first step right foot
LG: Chip NT with right arm, climb to MLB
C: Block NT
RG: Chip NT with left arm, climb to OLB
RT: Block DT, first step right foot
TE: Block DE, first step left foot
TH: Go in motion parallel to line of scrimmage, behind QB, on "ready," timed to reach QB on snap, receive handoff, run through 6 or 8 hole, whichever is better blocked
QB: Time snap for when TH reaches 5 or 3 hole, hand off to TH, fake handoff to FB running 3 hole
FB: First step left foot, fake carry through 3 hole
HB: Stalk block CB

ROCKET SERIES

Slots 33 Jet Fake

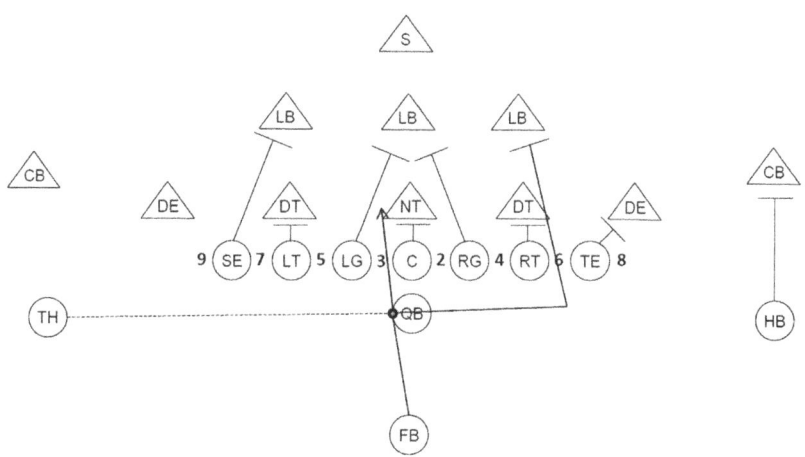

SE: First step left foot, block OLB
LT: Block DT, first step right foot
LG: Chip NT with right arm, climb to MLB
C: Block NT
RG: Chip NT with left arm, climb to MLB
RT: Block DT, first step right foot
TE: Block DE, first step left foot
TH: Go in motion parallel to line of scrimmage, behind QB, on "ready," timed to reach QB on snap, fake handoff, run through 6 or 8 hole
QB: Time snap for when TH reaches 5 or 3 hole, fake handoff to TH, hand off to FB running 3 hole
FB: First step left foot, receive handoff, carry through 3 hole
HB: Stalk block CB

ROCKET SERIES

Slots Jet Fake Option Left

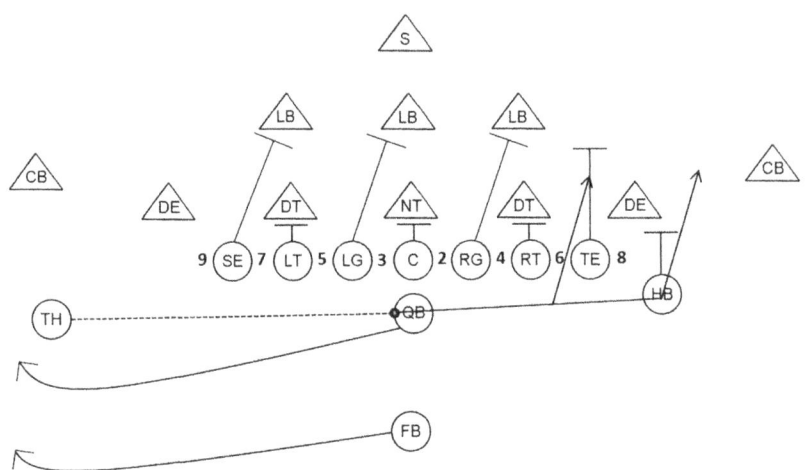

SE: First step left foot, block OLB
LT: Block DT, first step right foot
LG: Chip NT with right arm, climb to MLB
C: Block NT
RG: Chip NT with left arm, climb to OLB
RT: Block DT, first step right foot
TE: Block DE, first step left foot
TH: Go in motion parallel to line of scrimmage, behind QB, on "ready," timed to reach QB on snap, fake handoff, run through 6 or 8 hole
QB: Time snap for when TH reaches 5 or 3 hole, fake handoff to TH, run parallel to line of scrimmage, read DE to keep and cut back or pitch to FB
FB: First step left, get horizontal separation from QB, maintain 3-5 yard pitch relationship with QB as he runs parallel to line of scrimmage, hands ready to receive pitch based on CB read
HB: Block DE, first step right foot

ROCKET SERIES

Slots HB Slant Right

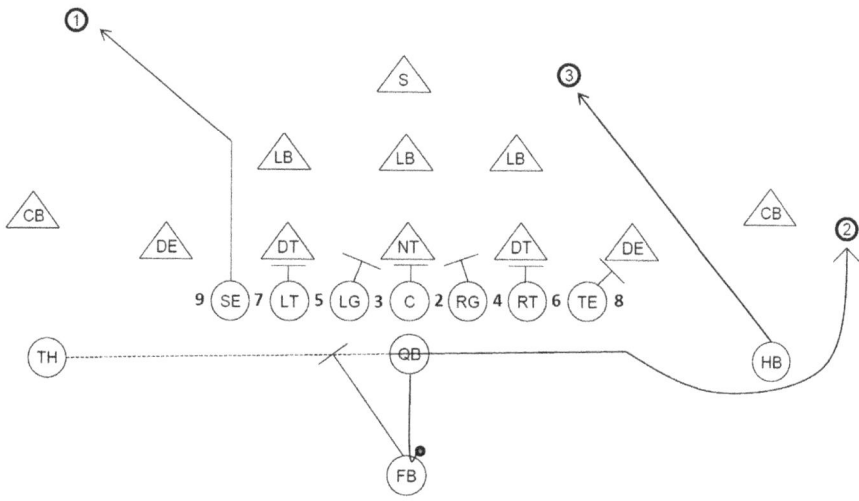

SE: First step right foot, run 5-yard corner route, cutting off right foot
LT: Pass block
LG: Pass block
C: Pass block
RG: Pass block
RT: Pass block
TE: Pass block
TH: Go in motion parallel to line of scrimmage, behind QB, on "ready," timed to reach QB on snap, fake handoff, run wheel route behind HB
QB: Time snap for when TH reaches 5 or 3 hole, fake handoff to TH, drop back five steps, set feet, throw to open receiver
FB: Pass block left
HB: First step left foot, run slant in front of CB

ROCKET SERIES

Slots 47 Jet Sweep

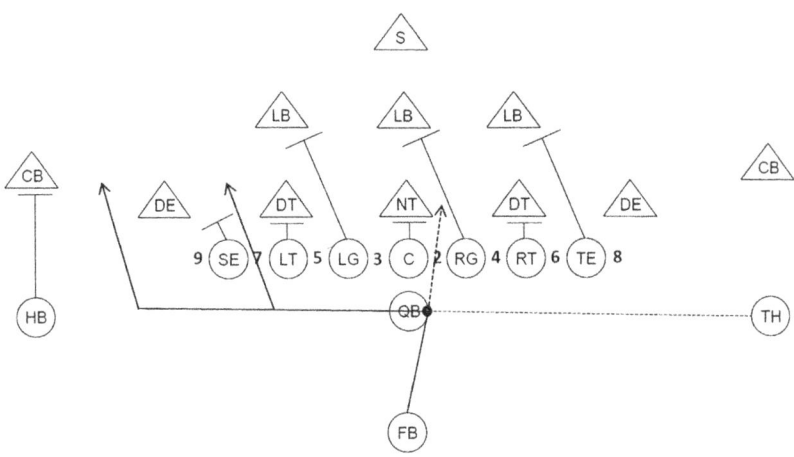

SE: Block DE, first step right foot
LT: Block DT, first step left foot
LG: Chip NT with right arm, climb to OLB
C: Block NT
RG: Chip NT with left arm, climb to MLB
RT: Block DT, first step left foot
TE: First step right foot, block OLB
TH: Go in motion parallel to line of scrimmage, behind QB, on "ready," timed to reach QB on snap, receive handoff, run through 7 or 9 hole, whichever is better blocked
QB: Time snap for when TH reaches 4 or 2 hole, hand off to TH, fake handoff to FB running 2 hole
FB: First step right foot, fake carry through 2 hole
HB: Stalk block CB

ROCKET SERIES

Slots 32 Jet Fake

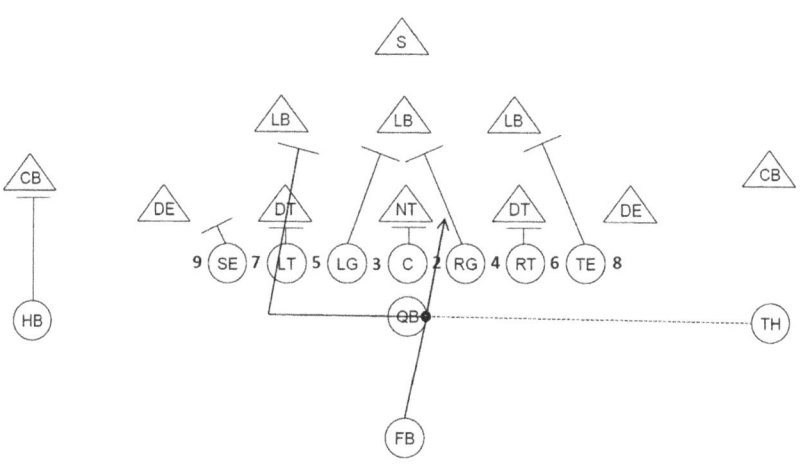

- **SE:** Block DE, first step right foot
- **LT:** Block DT, first step right foot
- **LG:** Chip NT with right arm, climb to MLB
- **C:** Block NT
- **RG:** Chip NT with left arm, climb to MLB
- **RT:** Block DT, first step left foot
- **TE:** First step right foot, block OLB
- **TH:** Go in motion parallel to line of scrimmage, behind QB, on "ready," timed to reach QB on snap, fake handoff, run through 7 or 9 hole
- **QB:** Time snap for when TH reaches 4 or 2 hole, fake handoff to TH, hand off to FB running 2 hole
- **FB:** First step right foot, receive handoff, carry through 2 hole
- **HB:** Stalk block CB

ROCKET SERIES

Slots Jet Fake Option Right

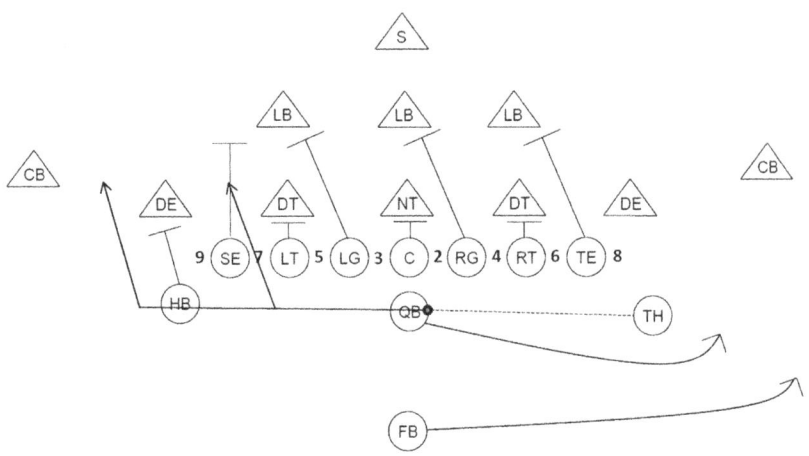

SE: First step left foot, block OLB
LT: Block DT, first step right foot
LG: Chip NT with right arm, climb to OLB
C: Block NT
RG: Chip NT with left arm, climb to MLB
RT: Block DT, first step right foot
TE: First step right foot, block OLB
TH: Go in motion parallel to line of scrimmage, behind QB, on "ready," timed to reach QB on snap, fake handoff, run through 7 or 9 hole
QB: Time snap for when TH reaches 4 or 2 hole, fake handoff to TH, run parallel to line of scrimmage, read DE to keep and cut back or pitch to FB
FB: First step right, get horizontal separation from QB, maintain 3-5 yard pitch relationship with QB as he runs parallel to line of scrimmage, hands ready to receive pitch based on CB read
HB: Block DE, first step left foot

ROCKET SERIES

Slots HB Slant Left

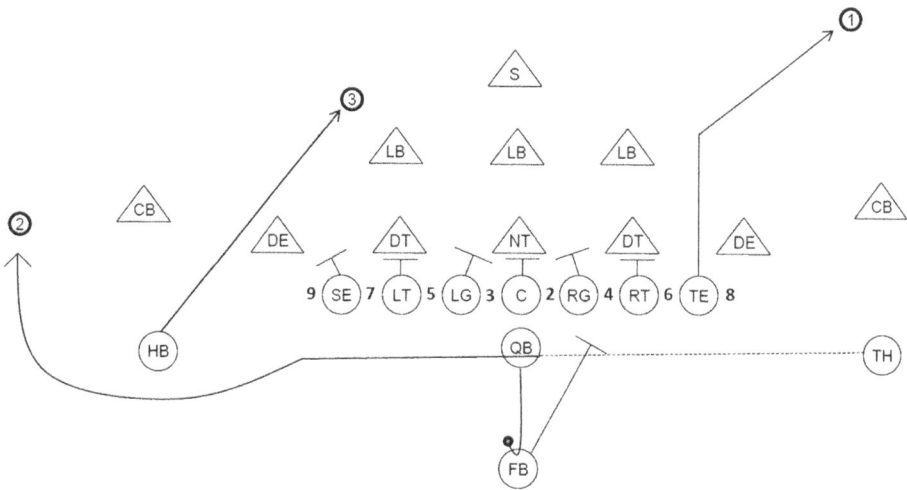

SE: Pass block
LT: Pass block
LG: Pass block
C: Pass block
RG: Pass block
RT: Pass block
TE: First step left foot, run 5-yard corner route, cutting off left foot
TH: Go in motion parallel to line of scrimmage, behind QB, on "ready," timed to reach QB on snap, fake handoff, run wheel route behind HB
QB: Time snap for when TH reaches 4 or 2 hole, fake handoff to TH, drop back five steps, set feet, throw to open receiver
FB: Pass block right
HB: First step right foot, run slant in front of CB

ROCKET SERIES

Slots Jet Fake TE Pass

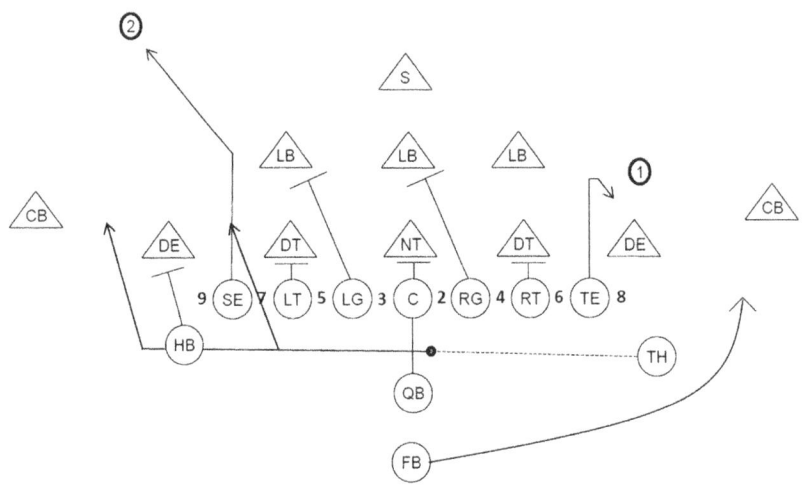

SE: First step right foot, run 5-yard corner, cutting off right foot
LT: Pass block
LG: Pass block
C: Pass block
RG: Pass block
RT: Pass block
TE: First step left foot, run 5-yard curl, settling outside OLB
TH: Go in motion parallel to line of scrimmage, behind QB, on "ready," timed to reach QB on snap, fake handoff, run through 7 or 9 hole
QB: Time snap for when TH reaches 4 or 2 hole, fake handoff to TH, drop back five steps, set feet, throw to open receiver
FB: First step right foot, run flare route right
HB: Pass block

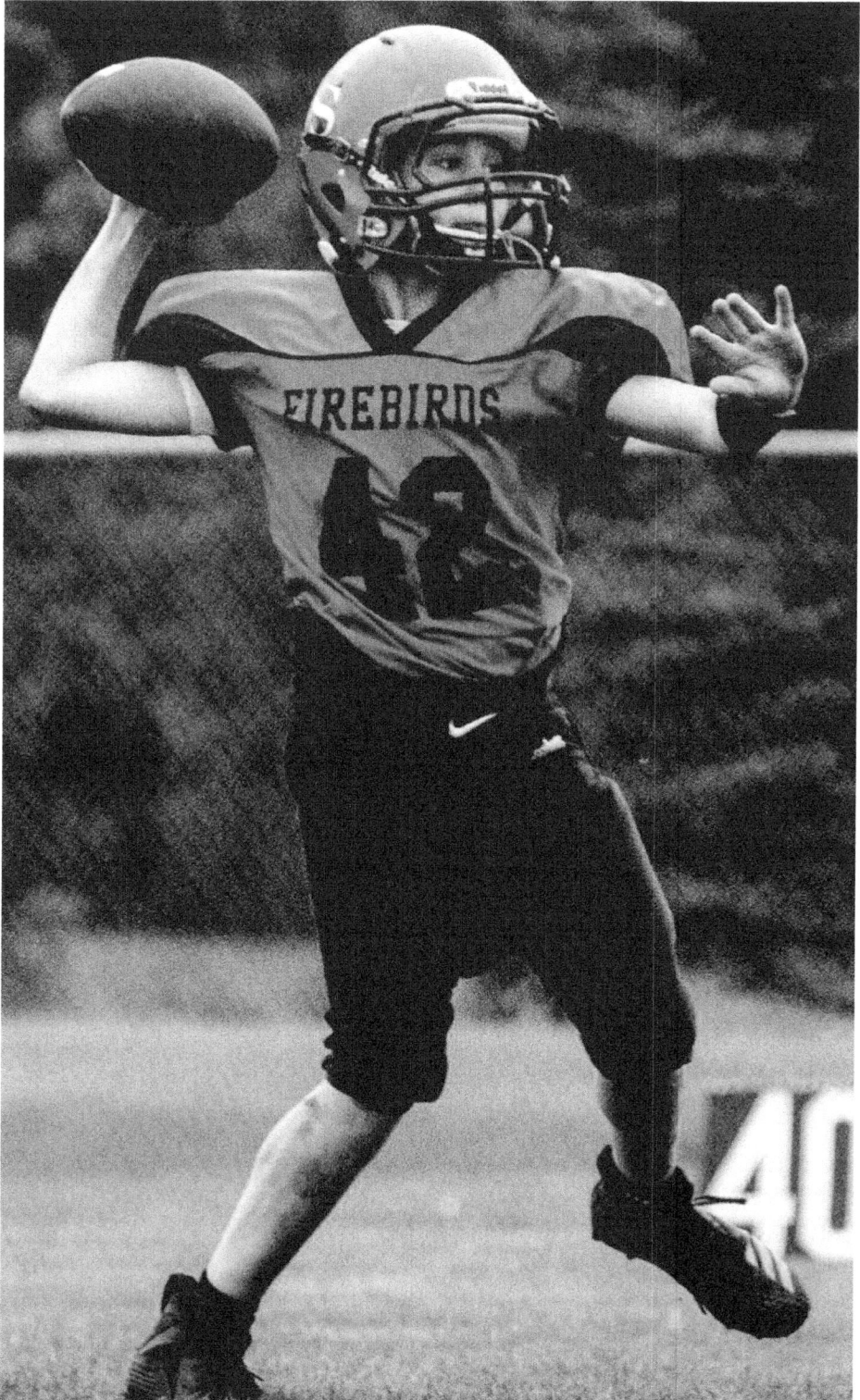

TWINS SERIES

Twins Right TH Fly

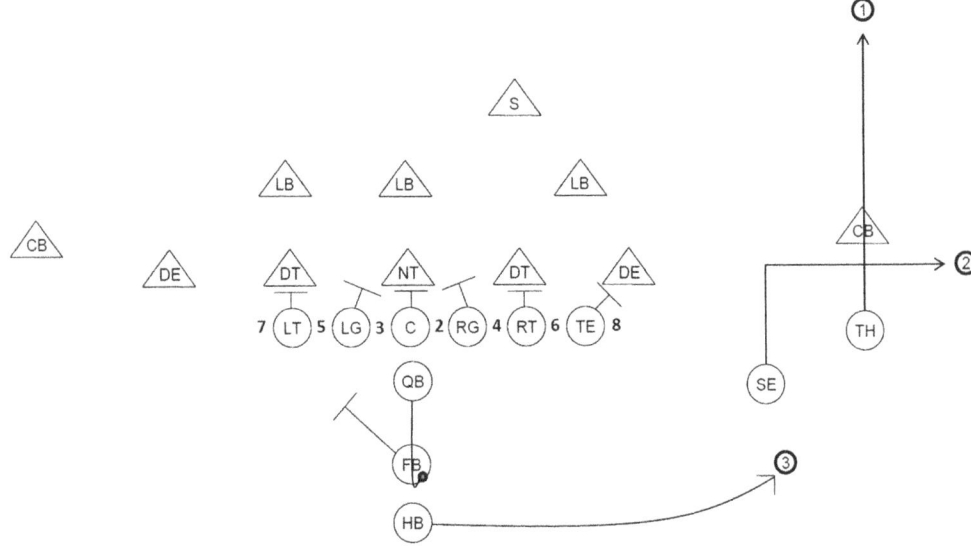

SE: Left foot first step, run 3-yard out, cutting off left foot
LT: Pass block
LG: Pass block
C: Pass block
RG: Pass block
RT: Pass block
TE: Pass block
TH: Left foot first step, run go route, snapping head over left shoulder after 10 yards
QB: 5-step drop, rolling slightly right, before setting feet and throwing to open receiver
FB: Pass block left
HB: Pass block right, flaring to flat if no pass rush threat

TWINS SERIES

Twins Left TH Fly

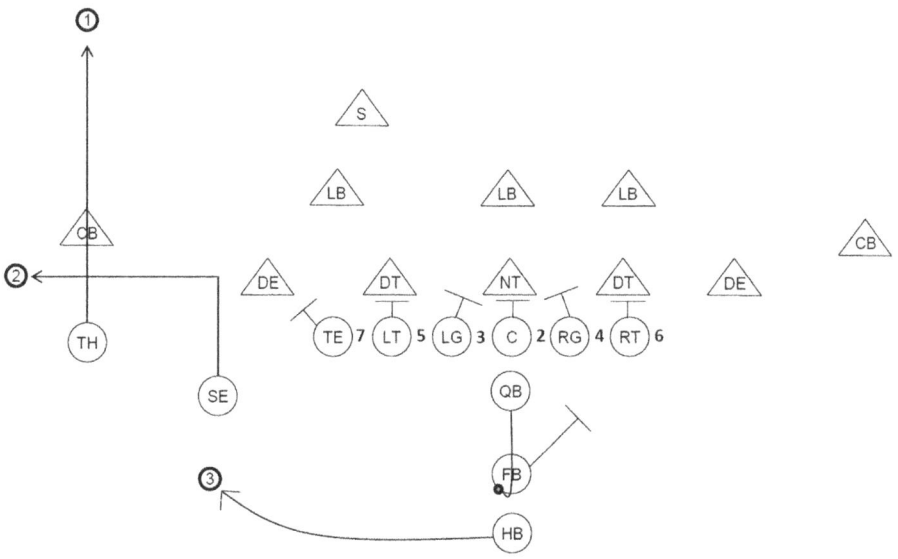

SE: Right foot first step, run 3-yard out, cutting off right foot
LT: Pass block
LG: Pass block
C: Pass block
RG: Pass block
RT: Pass block
TE: Pass block
TH: Right foot first step, run go route, snapping head over right shoulder after 10 yards
QB: 5-step drop, rolling slightly left, before setting feet and throwing to open receiver
FB: Pass block right
HB: Pass block left, flaring to flat if no pass rush threat

TWINS SERIES

Twins Right Smash

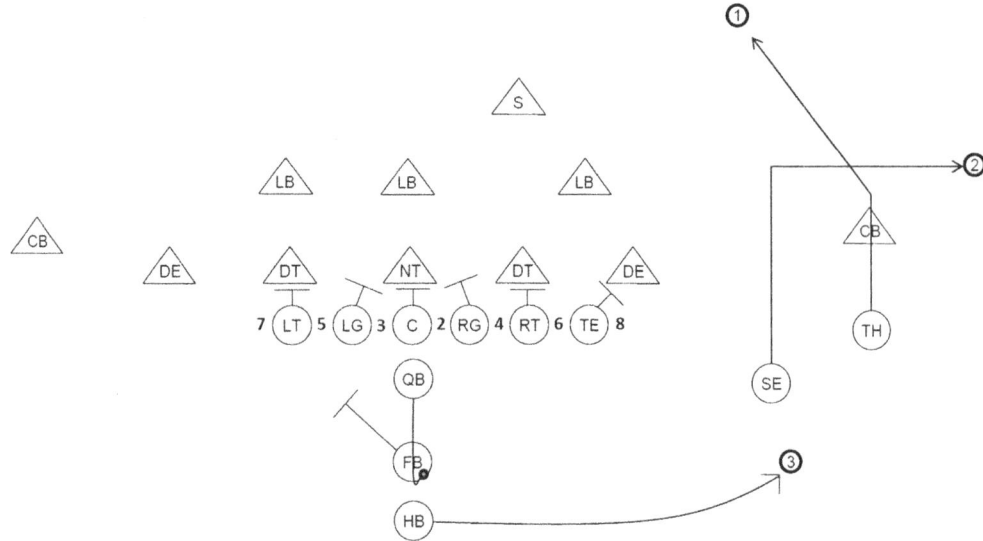

SE: Left foot first step, run 5-yard out, cutting off left foot
LT: Pass block
LG: Pass block
C: Pass block
RG: Pass block
RT: Pass block
TE: Pass block
TH: Left foot first step, run 5-yard post route, cutting off right foot
QB: 5-step drop, rolling slightly right, before setting feet and throwing to open receiver
FB: Pass block left
HB: Pass block right, flaring to flat if no pass rush threat

TWINS SERIES

Twins Left Smash

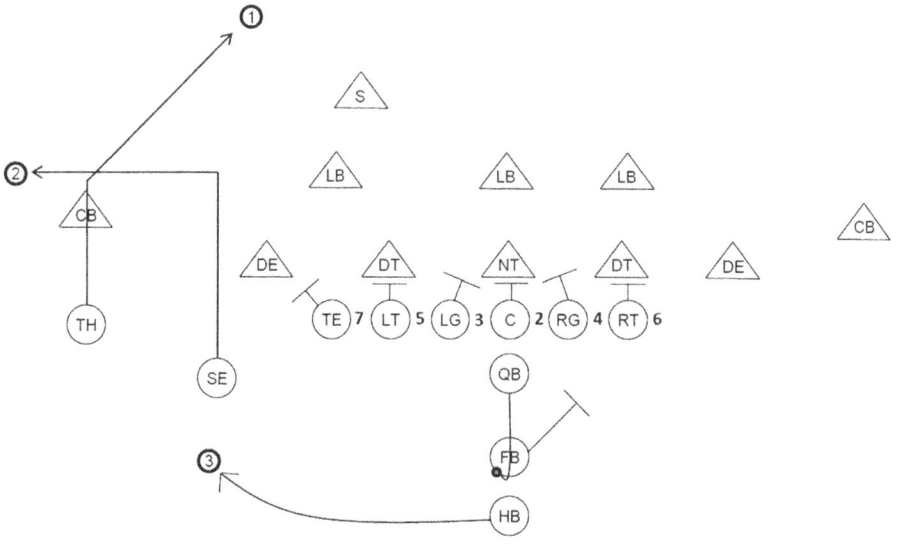

SE: Right foot first step, run 5-yard out, cutting off right foot
LT: Pass block
LG: Pass block
C: Pass block
RG: Pass block
RT: Pass block
TE: Pass block
TH: Right foot first step, run 5-yard post route, cutting off left foot
QB: 5-step drop, rolling slightly left, before setting feet and throwing to open receiver
FB: Pass block right
HB: Pass block left, flaring to flat if no pass rush threat

TWINS SERIES

Twins Right SE Corner

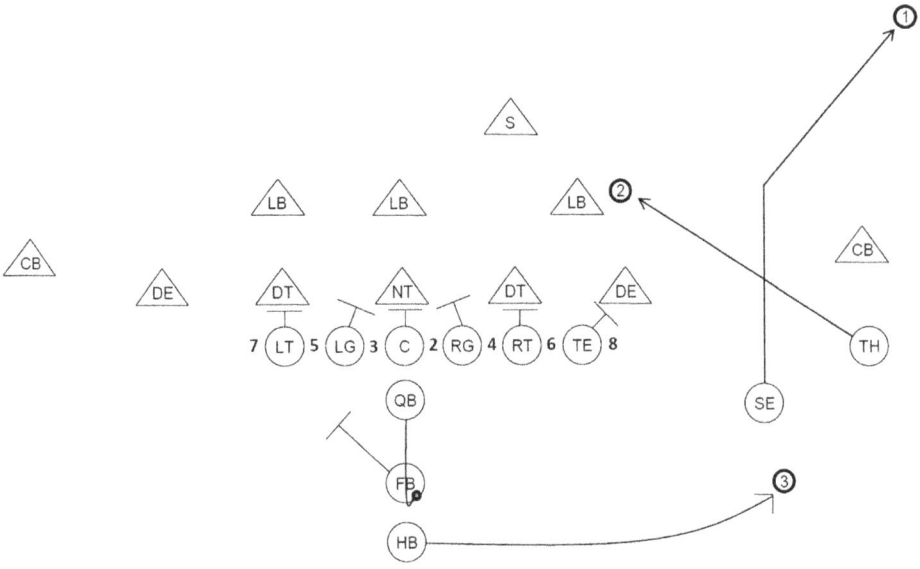

SE: Left foot first step, run 5-yard corner route, cutting off left foot
LT: Pass block
LG: Pass block
C: Pass block
RG: Pass block
RT: Pass block
TE: Pass block
TH: Right foot first step, run slant in front of CB
QB: 5-step drop, rolling slightly right, before setting feet and throwing to open receiver
FB: Pass block left
HB: Pass block right, flaring to flat if no pass rush threat

TWINS SERIES

Twins Left SE Corner

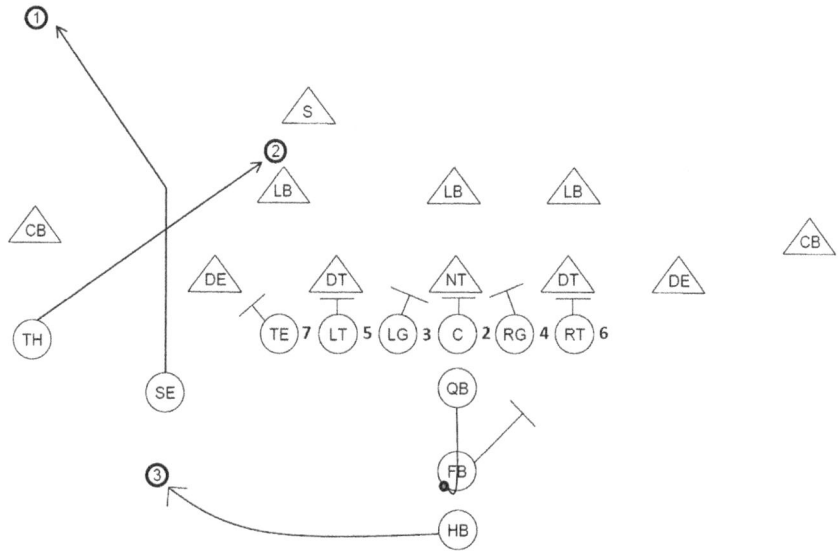

SE: Right foot first step, run 5-yard corner route, cutting off right foot
LT: Pass block
LG: Pass block
C: Pass block
RG: Pass block
RT: Pass block
TE: Pass block
TH: Left foot first step, run slant in front of CB
QB: 5-step drop, rolling slightly left, before setting feet and throwing to open receiver
FB: Pass block right
HB: Pass block left, flaring to flat if no pass rush threat

TWINS SERIES

Strong Right TE Corner

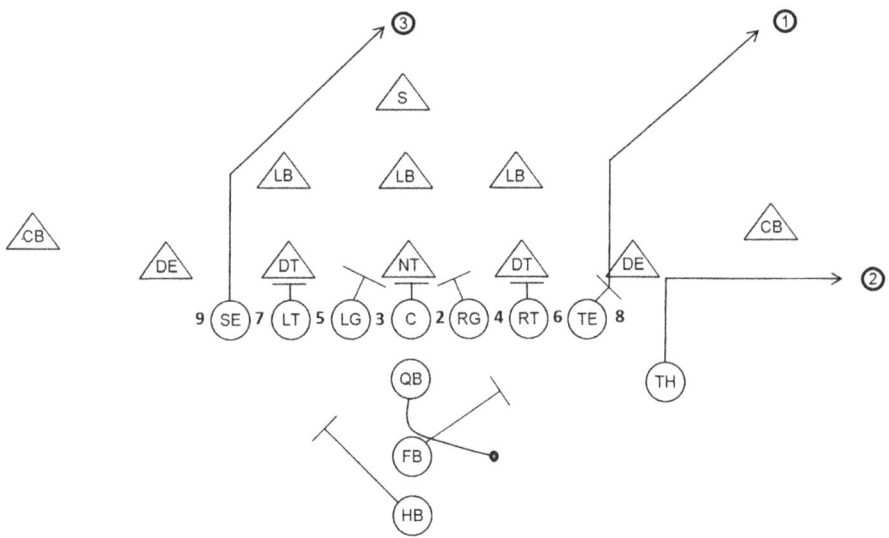

SE: Left foot first step, run 5-yard post route, cutting off left foot
LT: Pass block
LG: Pass block
C: Pass block
RG: Pass block
RT: Pass block
TE: Left foot first step, run 5-yard corner route, cutting off left foot
TH: Left foot first step, run shallow out route in front of CB
QB: 5-step drop, rolling slightly right, before setting feet and throwing to open receiver
FB: Pass block right
HB: Pass block left

TWINS SERIES

Strong Right TE Out

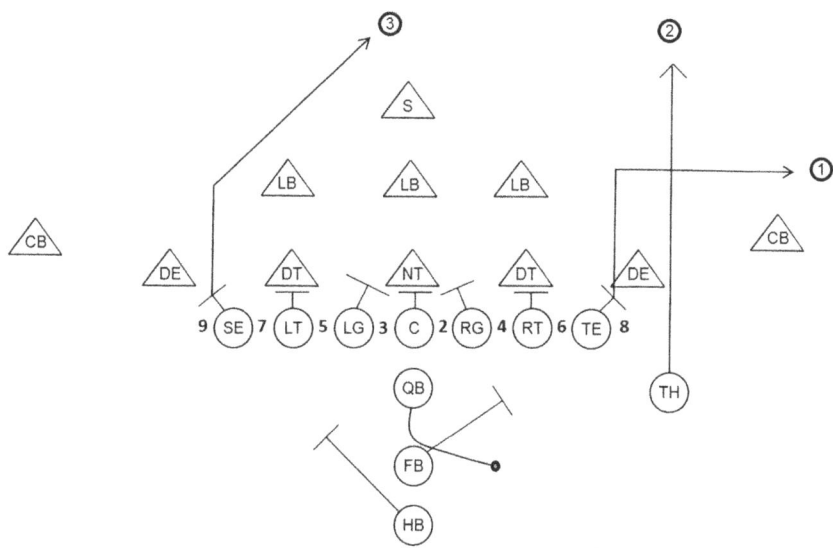

SE: Left foot first step, run 5-yard post route, cutting off left foot
LT: Pass block
LG: Pass block
C: Pass block
RG: Pass block
RT: Pass block
TE: Left foot first step, run 5-yard out route into space vacated by CB, cutting off left foot
TH: Left foot first step, run go route, snapping head over left shoulder after 10 yards
QB: 5-step drop, rolling slightly right, before setting feet and throwing to open receiver
FB: Pass block right
HB: Pass block left

TWINS SERIES

Strong Left TE Corner

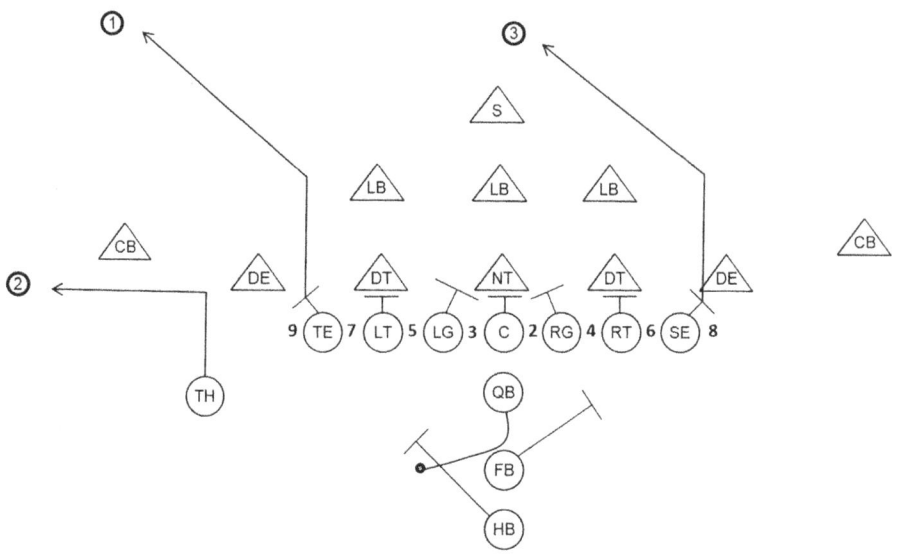

SE: Right foot first step, run 5-yard post route, cutting off right foot
LT: Pass block
LG: Pass block
C: Pass block
RG: Pass block
RT: Pass block
TE: Right foot first step, run 5-yard corner route, cutting off right foot
TH: Right foot first step, run shallow out route in front of CB
QB: 5-step drop, rolling slightly left, before setting feet and throwing to open receiver
FB: Pass block right
HB: Pass block left

TWINS SERIES

Strong Left TE Out

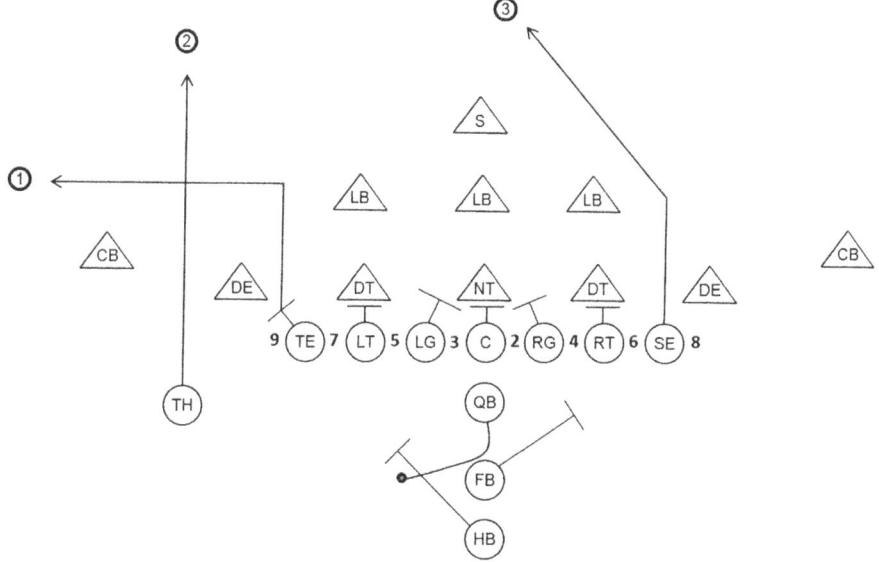

SE: Right foot first step, run 5-yard post route, cutting off right foot
LT: Pass block
LG: Pass block
C: Pass block
RG: Pass block
RT: Pass block
TE: Right foot first step, run 5-yard out route into space vacated by CB, cutting off right foot
TH: Right foot first step, run go route, snapping head over right shoulder after 10 yards
QB: 5-step drop, rolling slightly left, before setting feet and throwing to open receiver
FB: Pass block right
HB: Pass block left

TWINS SERIES

Gun Right TE Post HB Flat

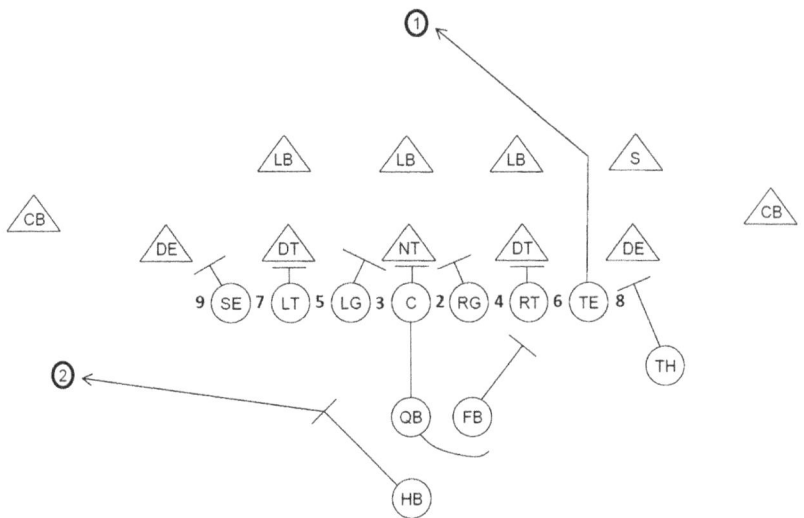

SE: Pass block
LT: Pass block
LG: Pass block
C: Pass block
RG: Pass block
RT: Pass block
TE: First step right foot, run 5-yard post route, cutting off right foot
TH: Pass block
QB: 5-step drop, rolling slightly right, before setting feet and throwing to open receiver
FB: Pass block right
HB: Pass block left, flaring to flat if no pass rush threat

TWINS SERIES

Gun Right TH Out and Up

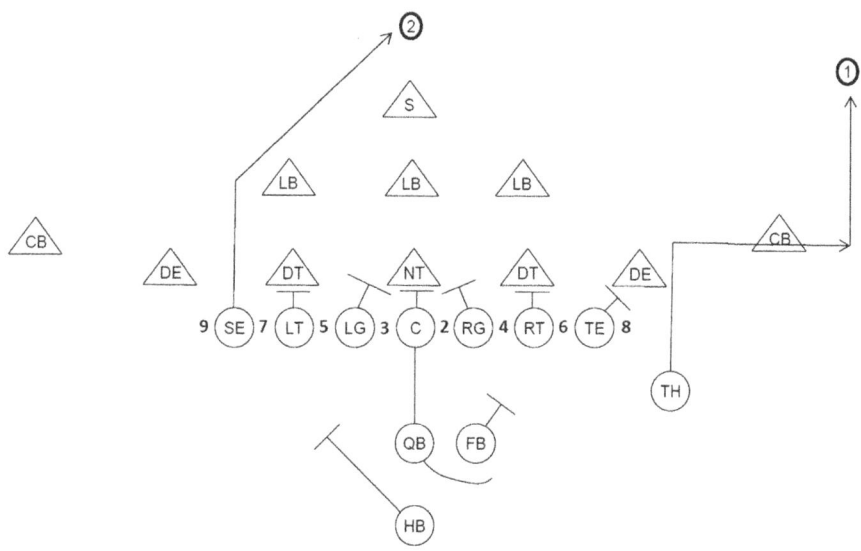

SE: First step left foot, run 5-yard post route, cutting off left foot
LT: Pass block
LG: Pass block
C: Pass block
RG: Pass block
RT: Pass block
TE: Pass block
TH: First step left foot, run out and up: 3-yard out, cutting off left foot, take three steps, then run go route, cutting off right foot, snapping head over left shoulder
QB: 5-step drop, rolling slightly right, before setting feet and throwing to open receiver
FB: Pass block right
HB: Pass block left

TRIPS SERIES

Trips Right Smoke Screen

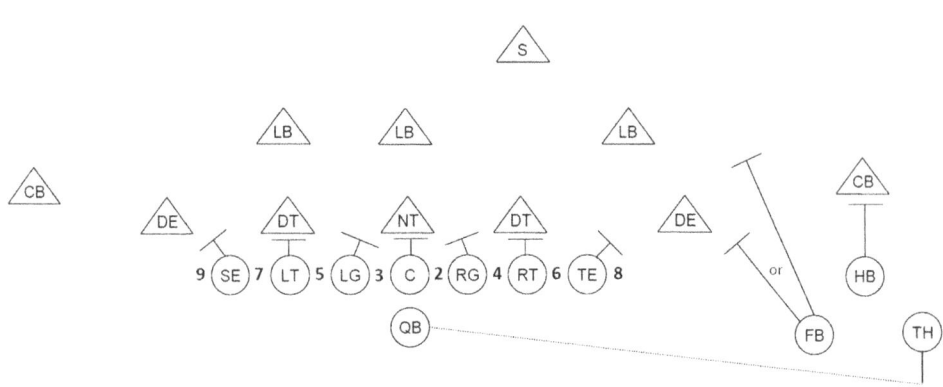

SE: Pass block
LT: Pass block
LG: Pass block
C: Pass block
RG: Pass block
RT: Pass block
TE: Pass block
TH: Left foot first step, take one step behind line of scrimmage, show hands, receive pass, cut off HB, FB blocks
QB: Receive snap, step right, throw to TH
FB: First step left foot, block DE or LB
HB: Stalk block CB

TRIPS SERIES

Trips Right Bubble Screen

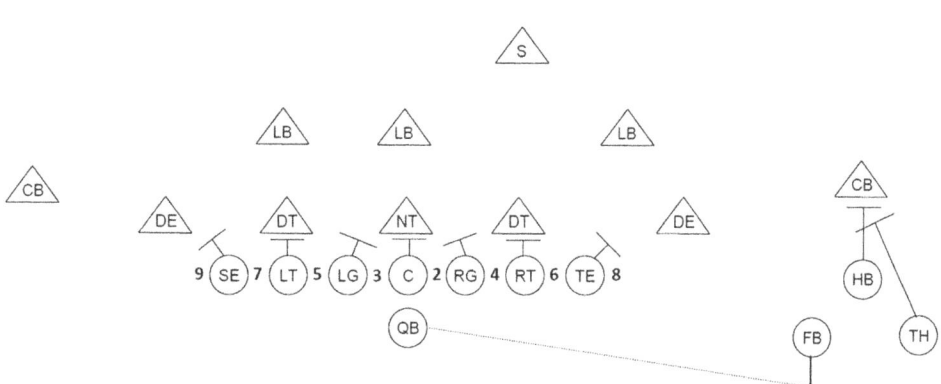

SE: Pass block
LT: Pass block
LG: Pass block
C: Pass block
RG: Pass block
RT: Pass block
TE: Pass block
TH: Stalk block CB
QB: Receive snap, step right, throw to FB
FB: Left foot first step, take one step behind line of scrimmage, show hands, receive pass, cut outside off HB, TH blocks
HB: Stalk block CB

TRIPS SERIES

Trips Left Smoke Screen

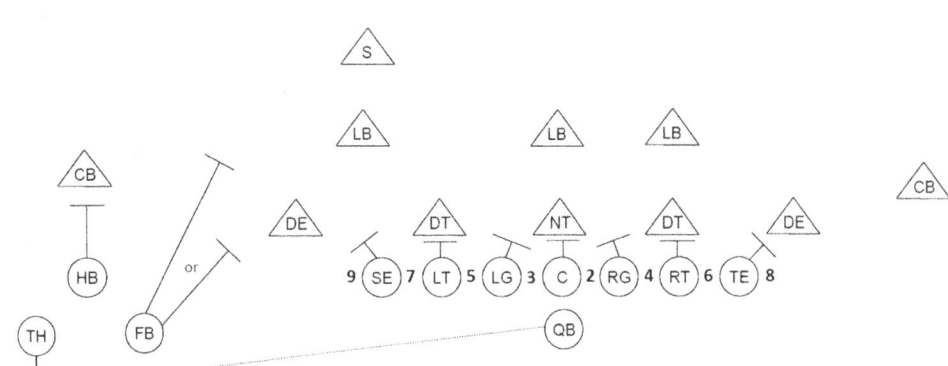

SE: Pass block
LT: Pass block
LG: Pass block
C: Pass block
RG: Pass block
RT: Pass block
TE: Pass block
TH: Right foot first step, take one step behind line of scrimmage, show hands, receive pass, cut off HB, FB blocks
QB: Receive snap, step left, throw to TH
FB: First step right foot, block DE or LB
HB: Stalk block CB

TRIPS SERIES

Trips Left Bubble Screen

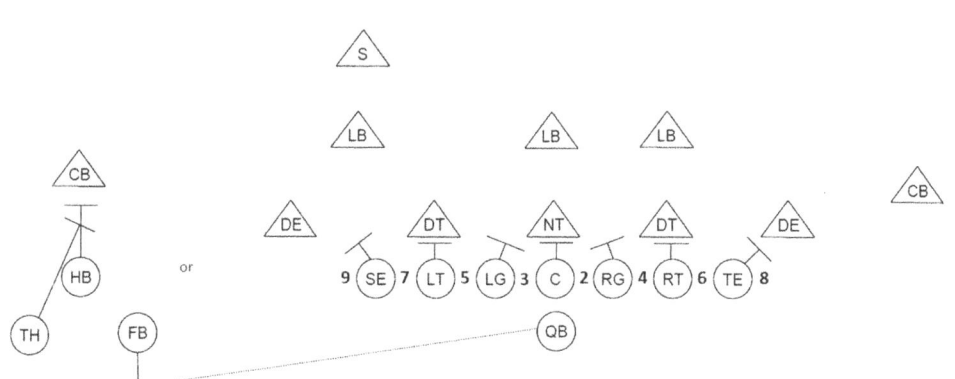

SE: Pass block
LT: Pass block
LG: Pass block
C: Pass block
RG: Pass block
RT: Pass block
TE: Pass block
TH: Stalk block CB
QB: Receive snap, step left, throw to FB
FB: Right foot first step, take one step behind line of scrimmage, show hands, receive pass, cut outside off HB, TH blocks
HB: Stalk block CB

TRIPS SERIES

Trips Right Bubble and Go

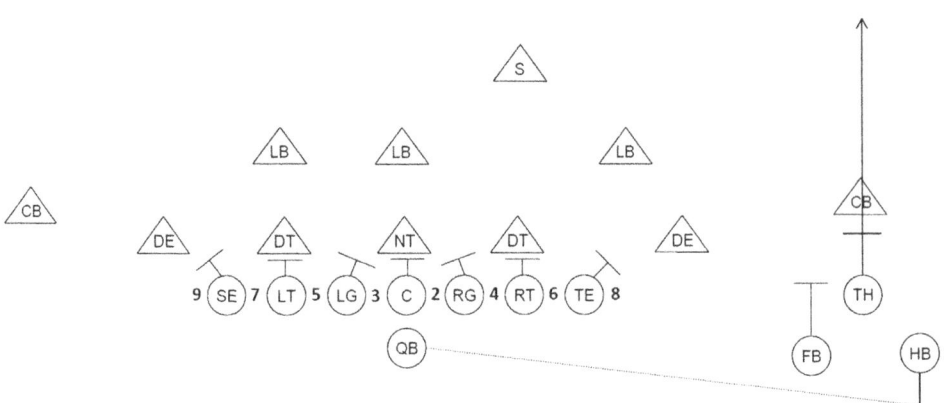

SE: Pass block
LT: Pass block
LG: Pass block
C: Pass block
RG: Pass block
RT: Pass block
TE: Pass block
TH: Fake stalk block CB, then run go route, snapping head over left shoulder after 10 yards
QB: Receive snap, step right, fake throw to FB, reset, throw to TH
FB: Fake block
HB: Left foot first step, take one step behind line of scrimmage, show hands as if intended target

TRIPS SERIES

Trips Left Bubble and Go

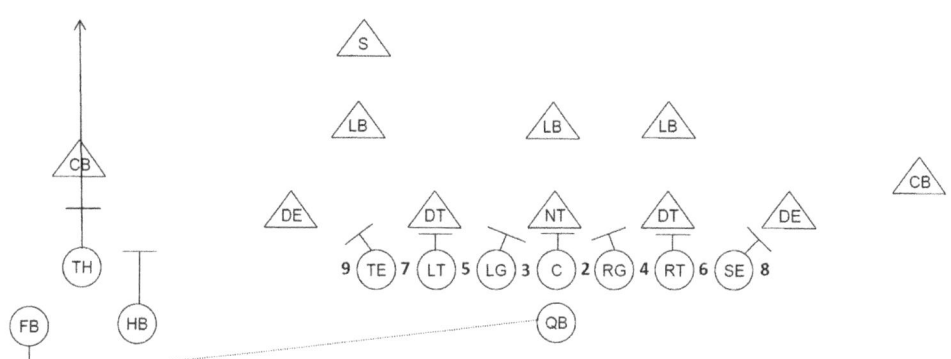

SE: Pass block
LT: Pass block
LG: Pass block
C: Pass block
RG: Pass block
RT: Pass block
TE: Pass block
TH: Fake stalk block CB, then run go route, snapping head over right shoulder after 10 yards
QB: Receive snap, step left, fake throw to FB, reset, throw to TH
FB: Right foot first step, take one step behind line of scrimmage, show hands as if intended target
HB: Fake block

TRIPS SERIES

Trips Right 12 Sneak

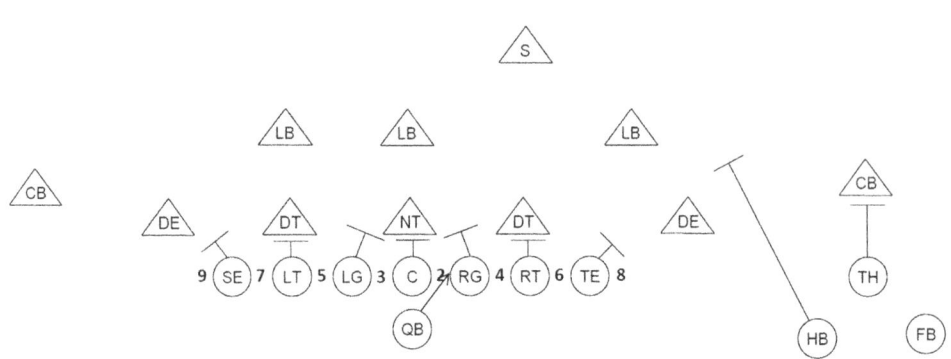

SE: Block DE, first step right foot
LT: Block DT, first step right foot
LG: Triple team NT with C
C: Block NT
RG: Triple team NT with C
RT: Block DT, first step left foot
TE: Block DE, first step left foot
TH: Block
QB: After receiving snap run through 2 hole off C right hip
FB: Block
HB: Block

TRIPS SERIES

Trips Left 13 Sneak

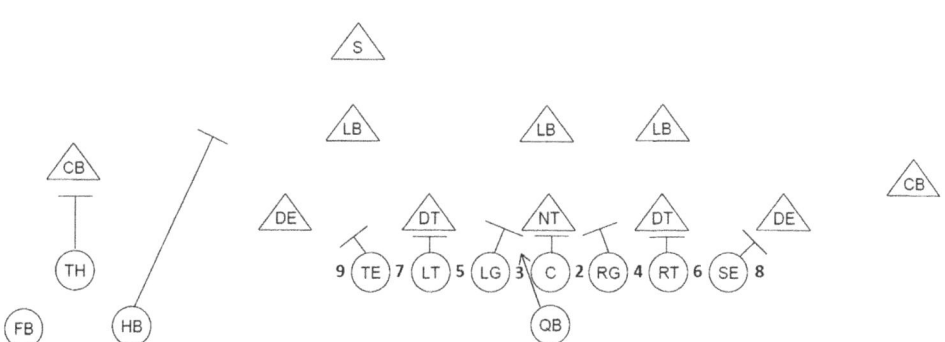

SE: Block DE, first step right foot
LT: Block DT, first step right foot
LG: Triple team NT with C
C: Block NT
RG: Triple team NT with C
RT: Block DT, first step left foot
TE: Block DE, first step left foot
TH: Block
QB: After receiving snap run through 3 hole off C left hip
FB: Block
HB: Block

EMPTY SERIES

Empty Curls

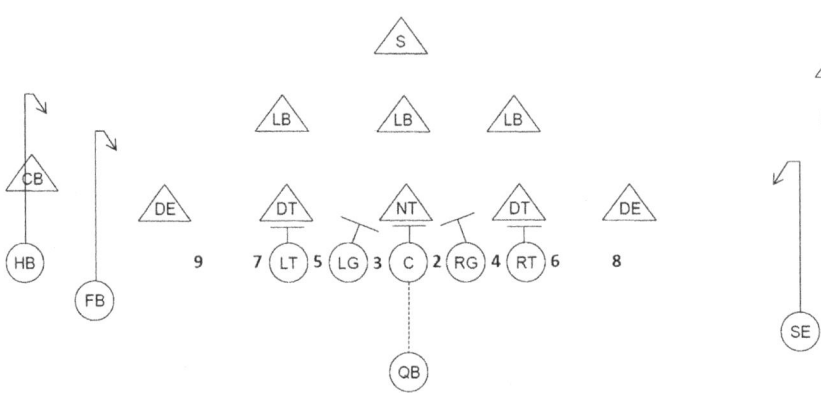

SE: First step left foot, 5-yard curl route, turning inside
LT: Pass block
LG: Pass block
C: Pass block
RG: Pass block
RT: Pass block
TE: First step left foot, 5-yard curl route, turning inside
TH: First step left foot, 5-yard curl route, turning inside
QB: Receive snap, throw to open receiver based on coverage
FB: First step right foot, 5-yard curl route, turning inside
HB: First step right foot, 5-yard curl route, turning inside

EMPTY SERIES

Empty Five Verticals

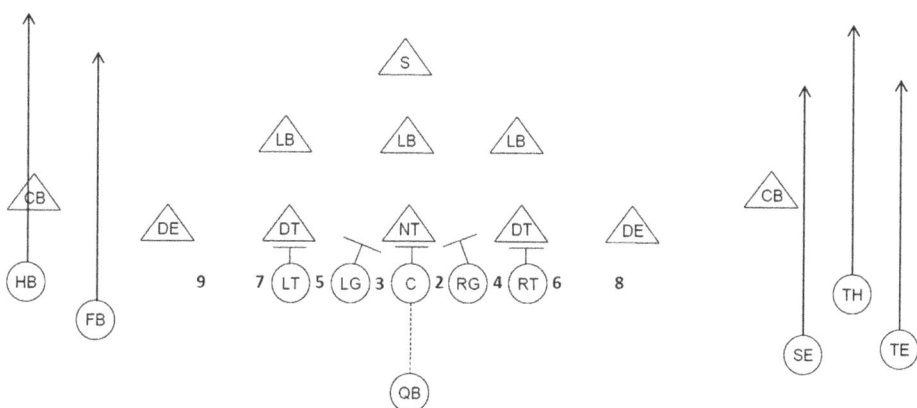

SE: First step left foot, run go route, snapping head over left shoulder after 10 yards
LT: Pass block
LG: Pass block
C: Pass block
RG: Pass block
RT: Pass block
TE: First step left foot, run go route, snapping head over left shoulder after 10 yards
TH: First step left foot, run go route, snapping head over left shoulder after 10 yards
QB: Receive snap, throw to open receiver based on coverage
FB: First step right foot, run go route, snapping head over right shoulder after 10 yards
HB: First step right foot, run go route, snapping head over right shoulder after 10 yards

EMPTY SERIES

Empty 52 Sneak

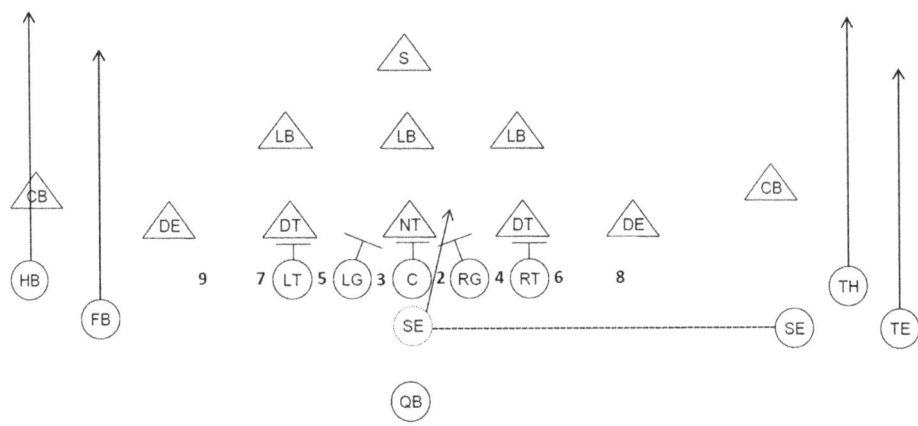

SE: Go in motion parallel to line on "down," stopping behind C, tap C on hip to activate silent snap
LT: Block DT, first step right foot
LG: Triple team NT with C
C: Block NT
RG: Triple team NT with C
RT: Block DT, first step left foot
TE: First step left foot, run go route
TH: First step left foot, run go route
QB: Fake receiving snap
FB: First step right foot, run go route
HB: First step right foot, run go route

EMPTY SERIES

Empty Draw

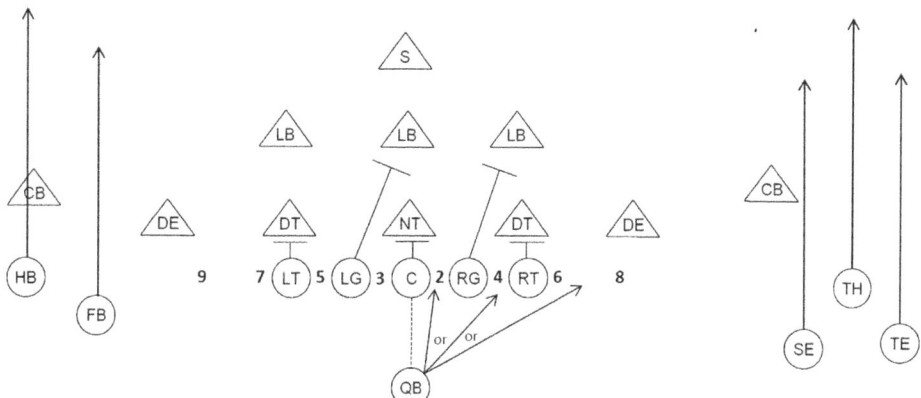

SE: First step left foot, run go route
LT: Block DT, first step right foot
LG: Chip NT with right arm, climb to MLB
C: Block NT
RG: Chip NT with left arm, climb to OLB
RT: Block DT, first step left foot
TE: First step left foot, run go route
TH: First step left foot, run go route
QB: Fake one step pass drop, then choose best running lane
FB: First step right foot, run go route
HB: First step right foot, run go route

HUDDLE

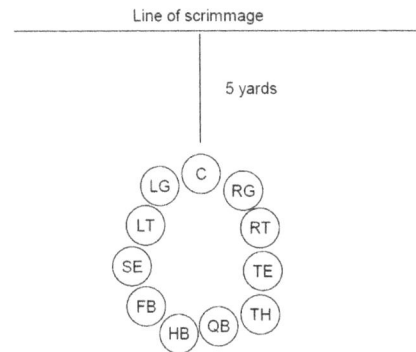

ROUTE TREE

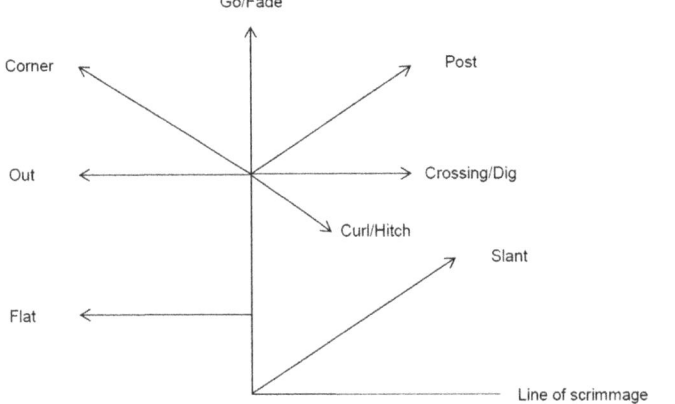

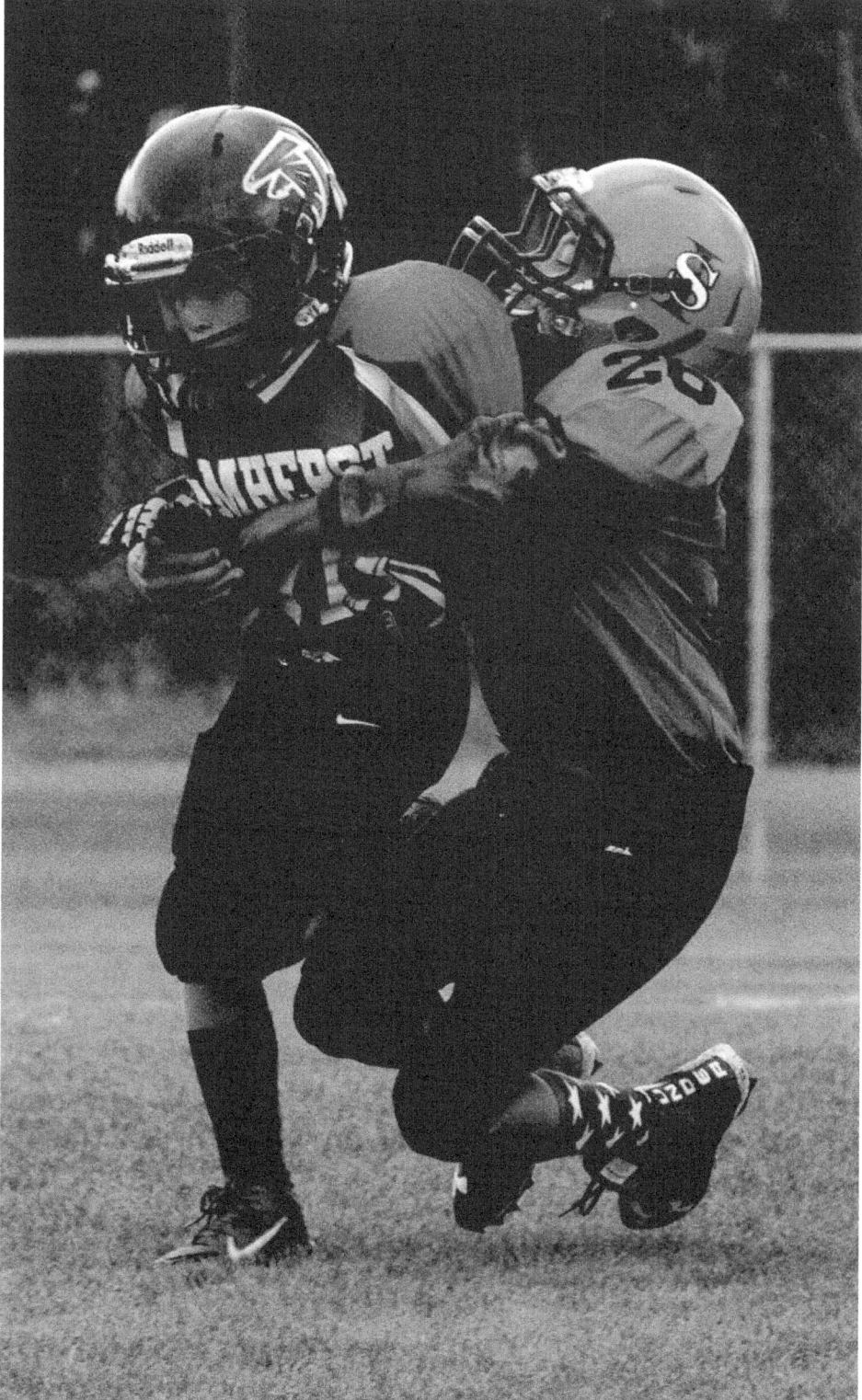

5-3 EAGLE

Defense

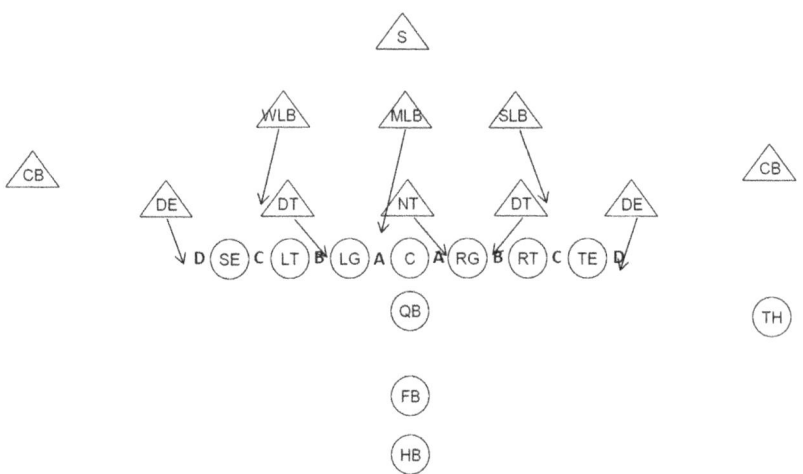

5-3 CRASH

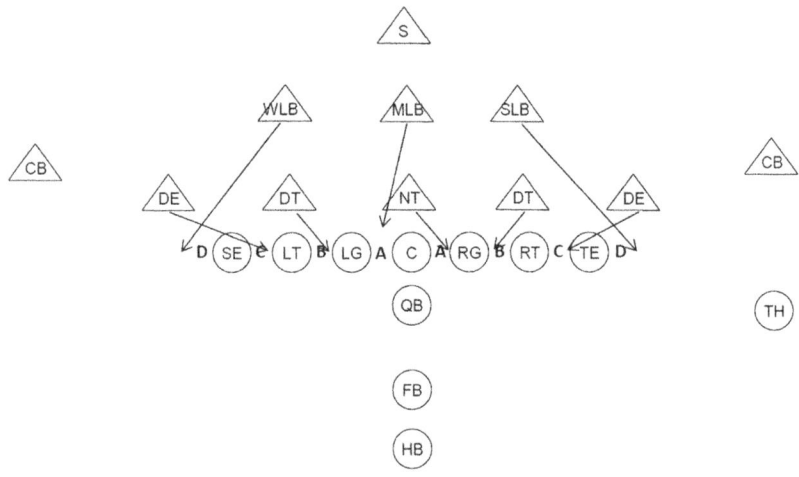

5-3 GOAL LINE

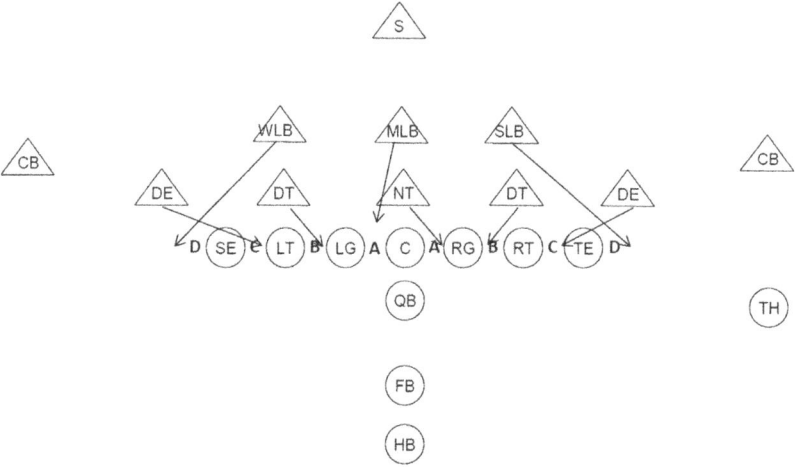

5-3 NICKEL

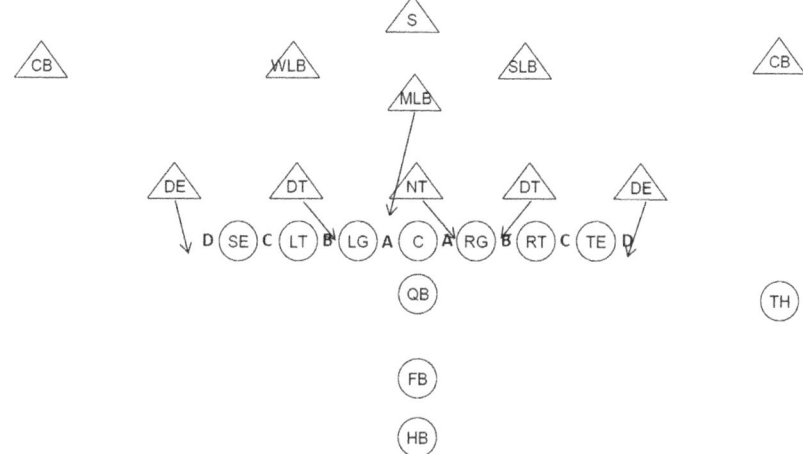

5-4 DEFAULT

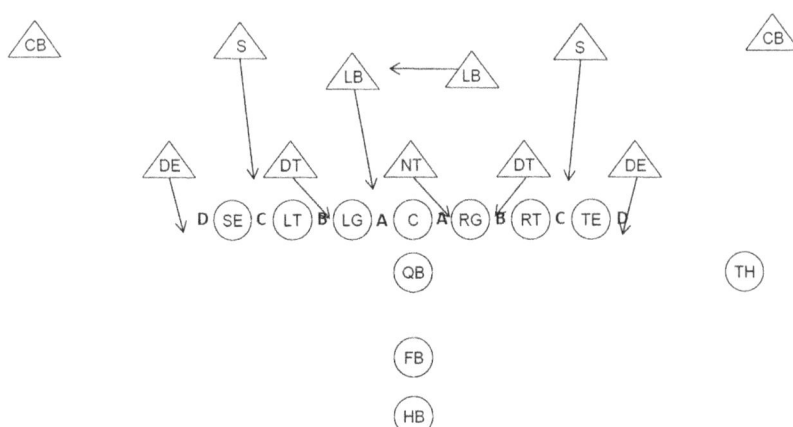

5-4 HULK

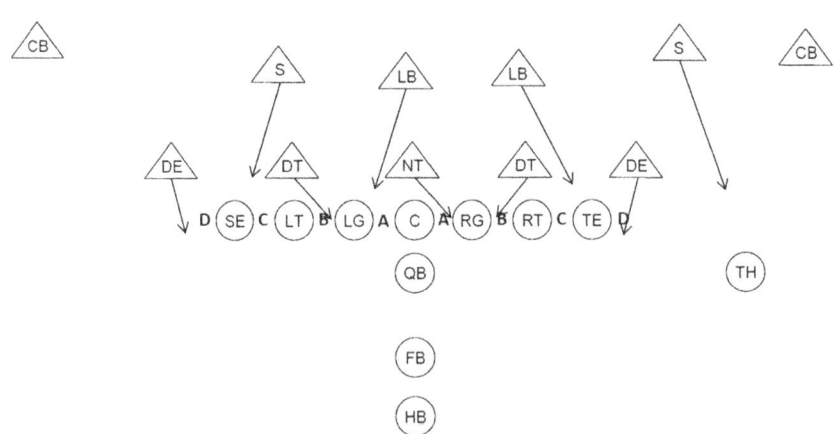

5-3 VS. TWINS

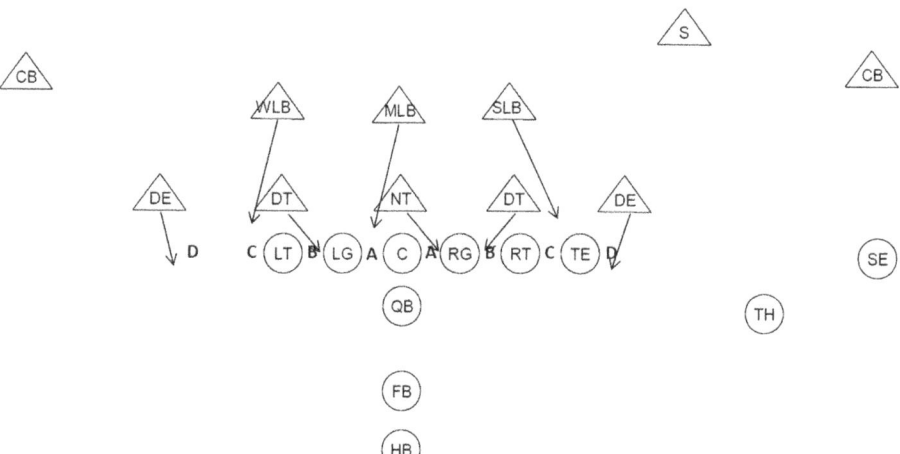

5-3 VS. TRIPS

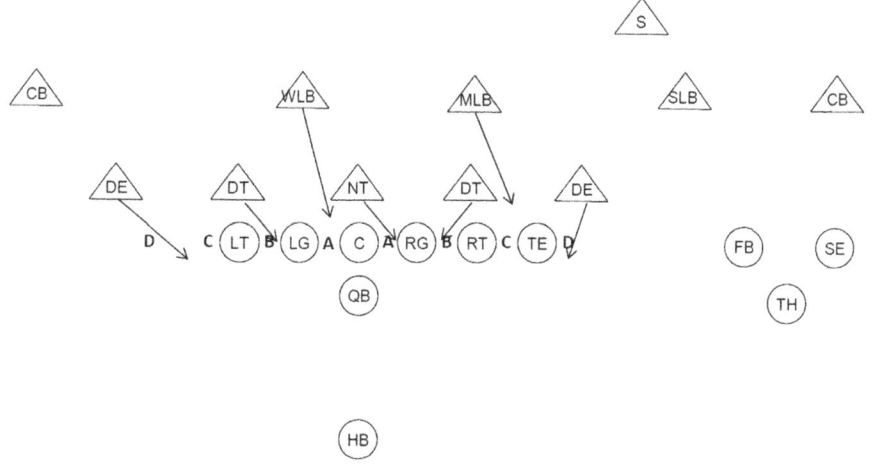

Special Teams

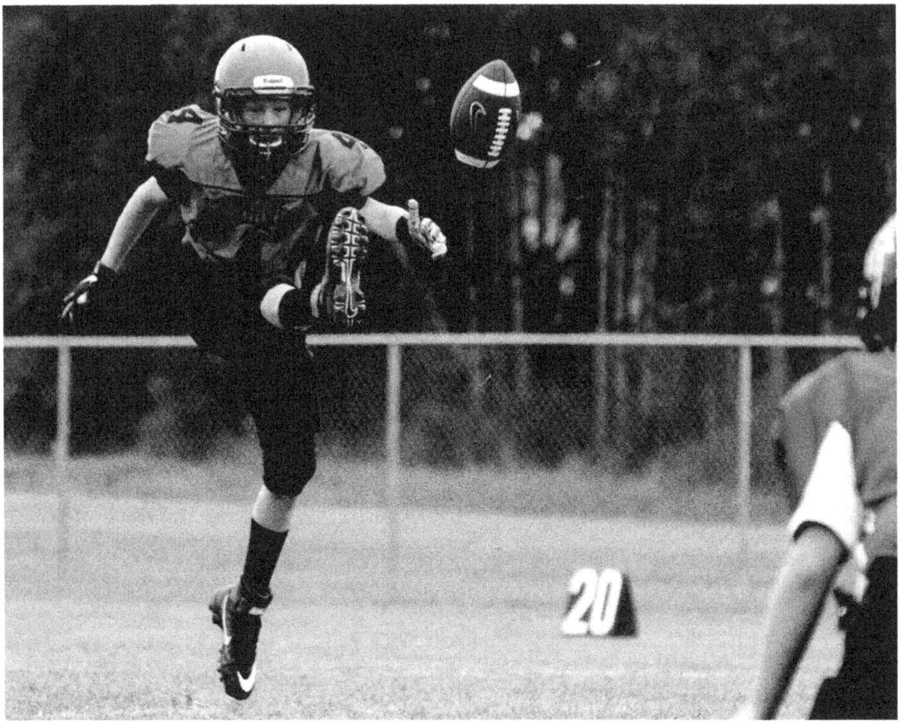

KICKOFF

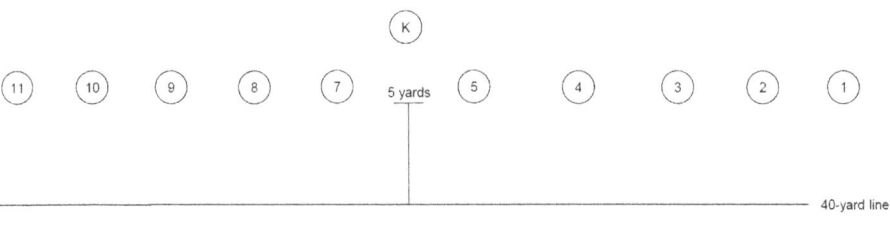

138   114 Youth Football Plays

KICKOFF RETURN

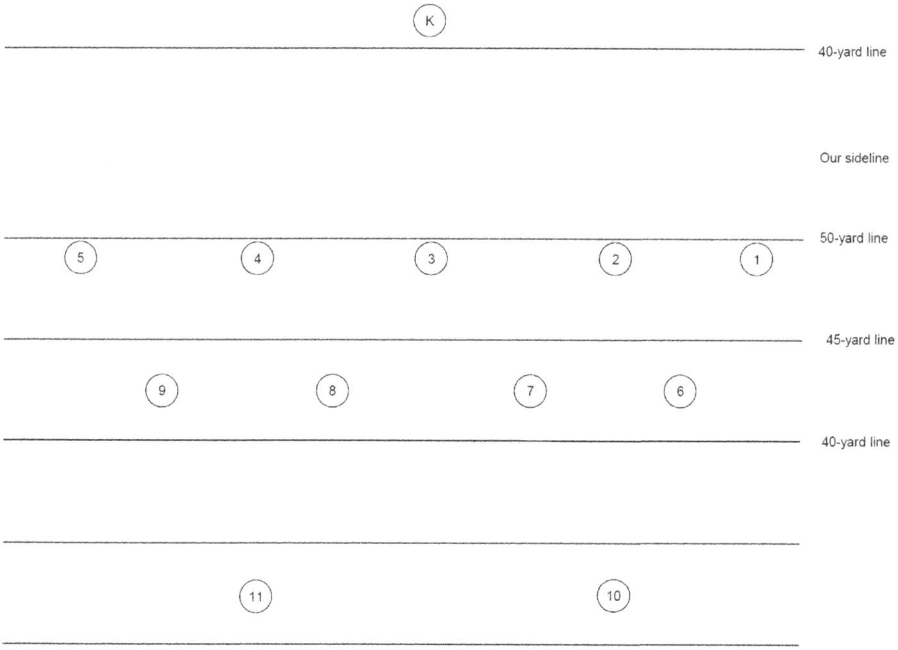

(K) — 40-yard line

Our sideline

(5)　(4)　(3)　(2)　(1) — 50-yard line

— 45-yard line

(9)　(8)　(7)　(6)

— 40-yard line

(11)　(10)

PUNT

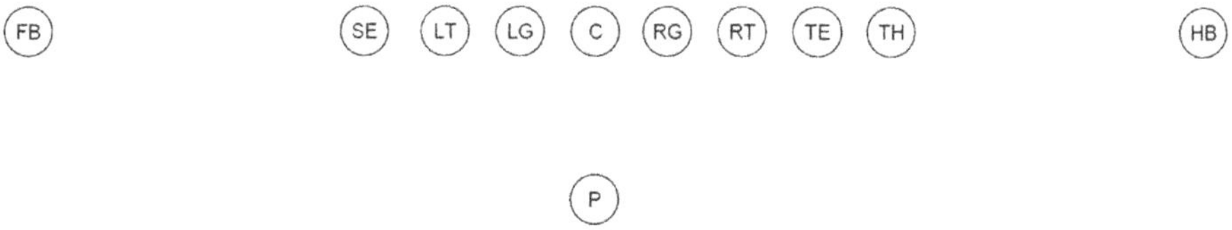

(FB)　(SE) (LT) (LG) (C) (RG) (RT) (TE) (TH)　(HB)

(P)

Scott Tappa **139**

PUNT RETURN

PLACEKICK

ALSO FROM THIS AUTHOR

First-Time Coach: Youth Football

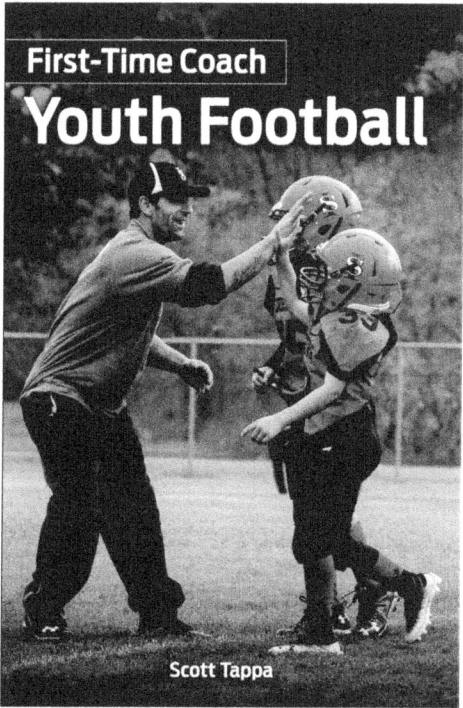

You have agreed to coach a youth football team.

You have enthusiasm, work ethic, charisma — and no experience. Where to start? In *First-Time Coach: Youth Football*, a veteran youth football coach takes you through the ins and outs of guiding a team. In these pages you will find guidance on preseason planning, preparing and running efficient practices, designing an offense and defense, managing your team on game day, and more. You will also find sample depth charts, call sheets, scouting forms, and practice planning templates. And if you need help coming up with an offense, we have included six runs and six passes to get you started. *First-Time Coach: Youth Football* will help you navigate this challenging, rewarding journey.

Made in the USA
Coppell, TX
26 November 2020